Dmytro Farina

Forward and Inverse Problems of Electrocardiography: Clinical Investigations

Vol. 4
Karlsruhe Transactions on Biomedical Engineering

Editor:
Universität Karlsruhe (TH)
Institute of Biomedical Engineering

Forward and Inverse Problems of Electrocardiography: Clinical Investigation

von
Dmytro Farina

universitätsverlag karlsruhe

Dissertation, Universität Karlsruhe (TH)
Fakultät für Elektrotechnik und Informationstechnik, 2008

Impressum

Universitätsverlag Karlsruhe
c/o Universitätsbibliothek
Straße am Forum 2
D-76131 Karlsruhe
www.uvka.de

Universitätsverlag Karlsruhe 2008
Print on Demand

ISSN: 1864-5933
ISBN: 978-3-86644-219-1

Forward and Inverse Problems of Electrocardiography: Clinical Investigations

Zur Erlangung des akademischen Grades eines

DOKTOR-INGENIEURS

von der Fakultät für

Elektrotechnik und Informationstechnik

der Universität Karlsruhe (TH)

genehmigte

DISSERTATION

von

M. Sc. Dmytro Farina
geb. in Krementschuk
Ukraine

Tag der mündlichen Prüfung: 5. Februar 2008
Hauptreferent: Prof. Dr. rer. nat. Olaf Dössel
Korreferent: Univ.-Prof. Dipl.-Ing. Dr. Bernhard Tilg

Contents

List of Figures

Chapter 1

Introduction

1.1 Motivation

Heart diseases are the principal cause of mortality in the modern society. Therefore it is highly important to improve the understanding of the functioning of the heart, which allows a physician to increase the efficiency of diagnostics and therapy as well as to reduce its costs.

Recording of an electrocardiogram (ECG) means the registration of changes of electric potential on the surface of the thorax. The form of ECG is defined by the electrical activity of the heart. Changes in the cardiac function immediately lead to changes in ECG. That is why ECG keeps its leadership in the everyday clinical practice as the main tool of noninvasive registration of cardiac activity.

A large work has already been done to classify the ECGs of patients with different heart disorders. This classification is essentially based on the empirical investigation of typical patterns; specific electrophysiological processes within the myocardium responsible for these patterns are usually left beyond detailed consideration.

Dealing with the relation between the cardiac activity (cause) and measured ECG (effect), two major types of problems show up. The forward problem of electrocardiography consists in the computation of an ECG from the given distributions of cardiac sources. These distributions can be measured (e.g. epicardial potentials recorded on the surface of the heart with a special sock containing a set of electrodes) or simulated employing a cardiac model.

The subject of the inverse problem is the reconstruction of cardiac sources from a given ECG. A large number of ECG channels is normally used, which increases the spatial resolution of this method. The inverse problem can be linear (e.g. for reconstruction of epicardial potentials or transmembrane voltages) or nonlinear (such as reconstruction of isochrons). In the present work only linear inverse problems are considered.

Another important task of this work is the correct modeling of cardiac activity. The optimization of the personalized cardiac model of a patient to fit his (or her) measured ECG can also be considered as a solution of the inverse problem. Such a model could provide valuable clinical information about the processes taking place in the heart of the patient and to forecast possible arrhythmias (e.g. fibrillation).

1.2 Structure of the Thesis

This work has the following structure. Chapters 2-5 are devoted to the state of the art in the field of cardiac modeling and the inverse problem of electrocardiography. In chapter 2 the medical background is considered. Chapter 3 provides a short description of modern methods of electrophysiological cardiac modeling. In chapter 4 it is described, how an ECG produced by a given cardiac model can be computed. Chapter 5 is devoted to the solution of the inverse problem of electrocardiography.

In chapters 6 and 7 the methodology of this work is described. Chapter 6 is devoted to the acquisition of the patient-specific data and the development of an anatomical model of the patient, as well as the processing of the ECG. In chapter 7 the development and customization of a personalized model of the patient's heart is considered.

Chapters 8 and 9 contain the results obtained in the course of this work. In Chapter 8 the modeling results are shown. Chapter 9 contains the reconstruction results obtained from the solution of the inverse problem.

The results are summarized and discussed in Chapter 10, in this chapter also the perspectives of the future work are described.

Chapter 2

Medical Background

2.1 Anatomy of the Heart

The human heart is a hollow organ located in the chest between the lungs behind the sternum. Its weight is typically between 250 and 300 g [12]. The walls of the heart consist of cardiac muscle tissue, the myocardium. The function of the heart is to pump the blood through the body, thus enabling the transportation of nutrient materials as well as oxygen to the organs.

The blood circulation system consists of two main parts. The pulmonary circulation carries the blood to the lungs, where it is saturated with oxygen. The systemic circulation is responsible for the transportation of blood saturated with oxygen throughout the body.

The anatomy of the heart is strongly connected with this structure of the circulation system [13]. The human heart is shown in figure 2.1. The two major chambers of the heart are the right and left ventricles. The right ventricle has a larger volume than the left one, but its walls are much thinner (around 4 mm). The right ventricle pumps the venous blood, which is poor with oxygen, through the pulmonary valve into the left and right pulmonary arteries. These arteries carry the blood to the lungs, where the blood is saturated with oxygen. Afterwards the blood is passing through the left atrium and reaches the left ventricle. The left ventricle has a relatively thick wall (normally about 10 mm in the diastolic phase [14]), thus producing a high pressure of around 140 mmHg. It is responsible for pumping of arterial blood, which is rich with oxygen, throughout the body.

Each ventricle has an atrium, a smaller chamber that works as a secondary pump to fill up the ventricle with blood. The atria are separated from the ventricles with the mitral (left) and tricuspid (right) valves, which prevent the inversion of the blood flow. The valves are supported with papillary muscles.

The coronary vessels supply the ventricular myocardium with blood. An interruption of the blood inflow results in the damage of myocardial tissue due to the oxygen shortage, thus causing myocardial infarction [15].

The anisotropy of ventricular myocardium is caused by the prolate form of individual myocytes, which are interconnected into an oriented structure (see figure 2.2). The fiber orientation is defined mainly by the *helix angle* – the angle between the fiber orientation

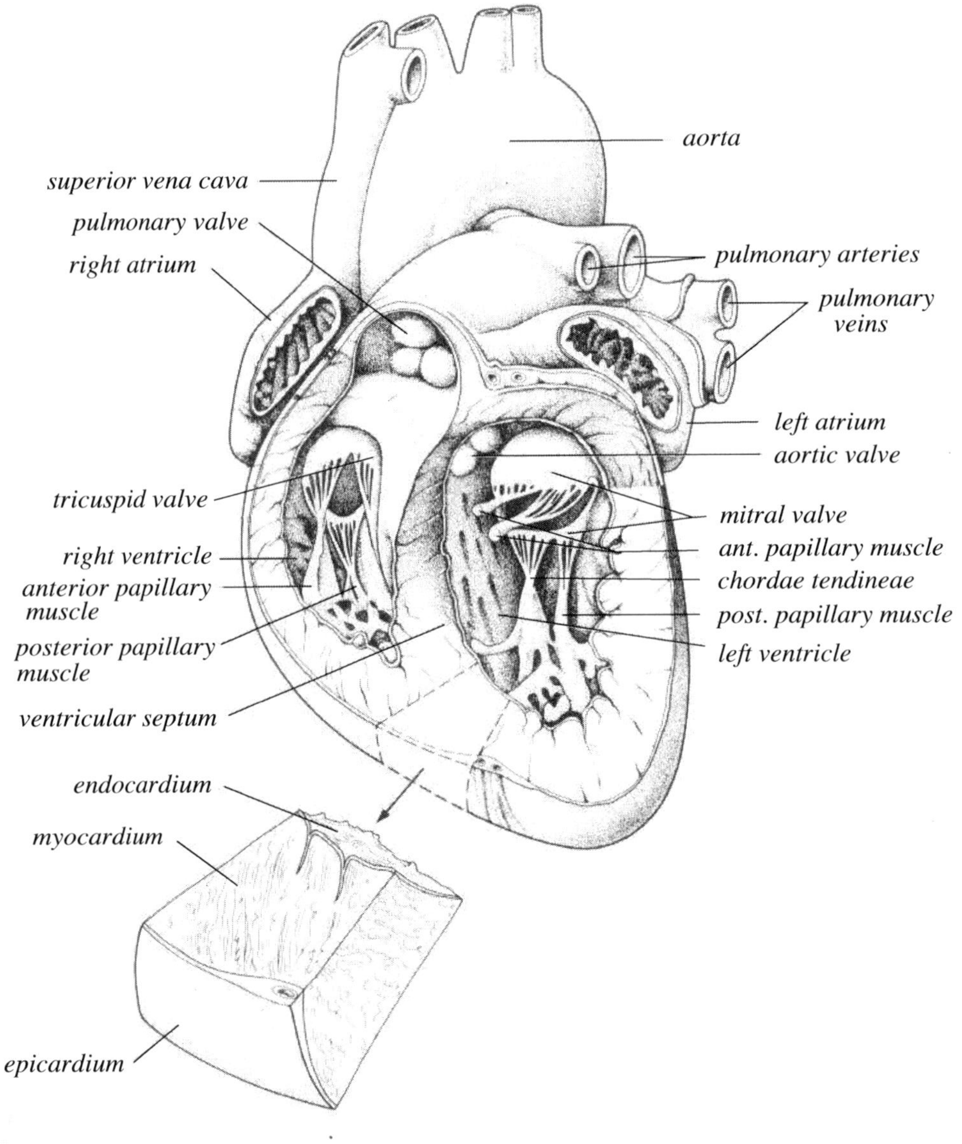

Figure 2.1: Anatomy of the heart [1]

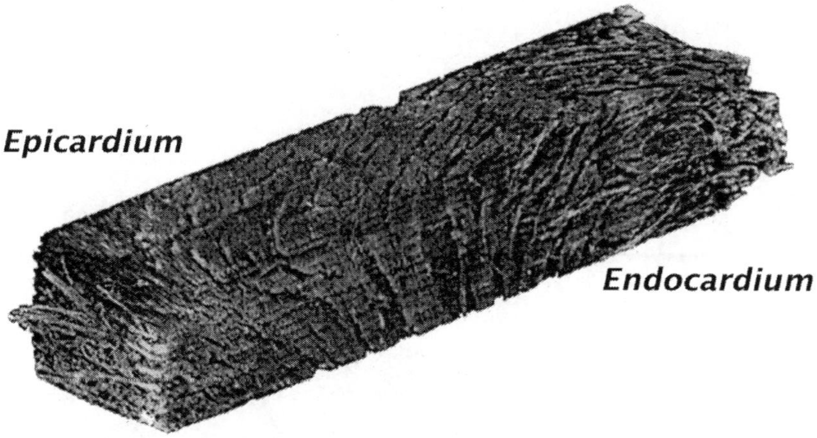

Figure 2.2: *Crossection of the ventricular wall of a rat. The fiber twist is clearly visible [2].*

and equatorial direction of the heart in a plain parallel to the endocardial surface (α_1 in figure 2.3).

According to the measurements of Streeter in [16, 3], in the human left ventricle the helix angle changes from $+55°$ in the subendocardial layer to $-75°$ in the subepicardial tissue. Also the electrophysiological properties of myocardial cells are changing across the ventricular wall – see section 2.3.

2.2 Electrophysiology of the Heart

The heart contains two types of muscle cells: those producing and transferring the electrical excitation as well as those reacting on the excitation with contraction [17]. The excitation triggering the cardiac contraction is generated within the heart, thus assuring an autonomous heart function.

The activation is normally generated in the sinoatrial node (SA-node), afterwards propagating through both atria to the atrioventricular node (AV-node). The AV-node acts as a secondary pacemaker if the SA-node does not function or its impulses are blocked. Afterwards the excitation conduction system (right and left Tawara bundles as well as Purkinje fibers) carries the excitation to the ventricular myocardium. All sections of the excitation conduction system possess the ability to generate the excitation, but the frequency of this autorhythmia is much smaller than that of the sinus node.

The myocytes forming the atrial and ventricular myocardium are coupled through gap junctions, thus being able to transfer the activation from cell to cell. Therefore the excitation appearing somewhere in the heart can be transferred throughout the myocardium leading to the contraction of the whole heart (the so-called "all-or-nothing" contraction).

The electrophysiological state of myocardial cells is characterized by their transmem-

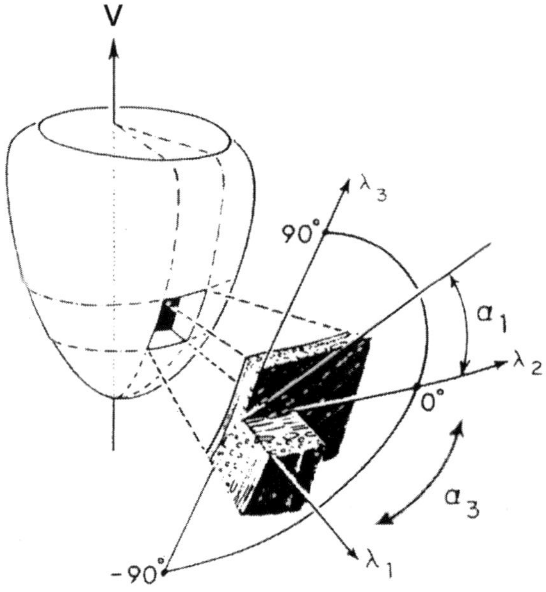

Figure 2.3: *Definition of helix angle* α_1 *defining the fiber orientation in the ventricle wall [3].*

brane voltage (TMV), meaning the potential difference between the intra- and extracellular spaces:

$$V_m = \varphi_i - \varphi_e. \tag{2.1}$$

At rest the TMV of the myocytes is equal to $-80\ mV$. Once the activation front arrives, the flow of different ions through the cell membrane leads to the rapid change of the TMV up to $+20\ mV$. The activation propagation throughout the ventricles corresponds to the QRS-complex of ECG. After the depolarization follows the plateau phase, which means that the TMV stays more or less constant. During this phase the mechanical contraction of the heart takes place. Afterwards the repolarization phase comes, during which the TMV changes back to $-80\ mV$. This phase is reproduced by the T-wave of ECG. After the electrical relaxation follows also the mechanical relaxation of the heart.

The change in TMV after the activation of excitable cell is called *action potential.* Different tissues of the heart possess different action potential curves. A short summary on the forms of action potential as well as the sequence of cardiac activation is shown in figure 2.4.

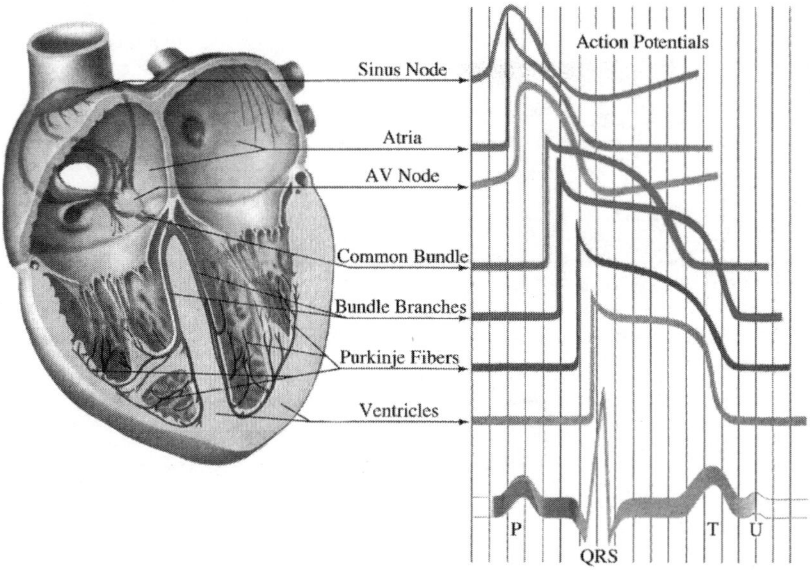

Figure 2.4: *Action potential curves in different tissues of the heart. The segments of the ECG curve defined by each cardiac tissue are shown with corresponding colors [4].*

2.3 Dispersion of Action Potential Duration

The T-wave represents the relaxation phase of the cardiac cycle. Its form is defined mostly by the inhomogeneity of the action potential duration (APD) within the myocardium. The transmural dispersion, the base-apex dispersion as well as the interventricular dispersion of the APD within the myocardium are mostly considered [18].

The transmural heterogeneity of the APD has already been well studied [19, 20, 5]. Three different cell types are recognized within the ventricular wall: epicardial, midmyocardial (M-cells) and endocardial cells. The M-cells possess the longest APD of about 420 ms, whereas the APD for the endo- and epicardial cells is significantly shorter (about 290 ms, see figure 2.5) [5]. The electrical coupling of the cells decreases this dispersion [21], a further decrease can be caused by several anesthetics [20]. This kind of dispersion has been reproduced by various myocardial cell models [22, 23].

The base-apex APD dispersion has been detected for different mammalian hearts, such as dogs [24], guinea pigs [25], pigs [26] etc. The APD gradient orientation was different for different species. In the case of guinea pigs the apex to base APD dispersion has been shown to decrease with the increasing heart rate [27].

APD dispersion of left vs. right ventricle of the canine heart has not been detected, but still the I_{to1}-mediated action potential notch is larger in the right ventricular epicardium than in the left one [28]. In [29] the I_{to1} and I_{Ks} currents are also shown to be larger in right than in left ventricular M-cells. These currents are normally responsible for the decrease of APD. It also follows from [5] and [30], that human mean epicardial I_{to} in the

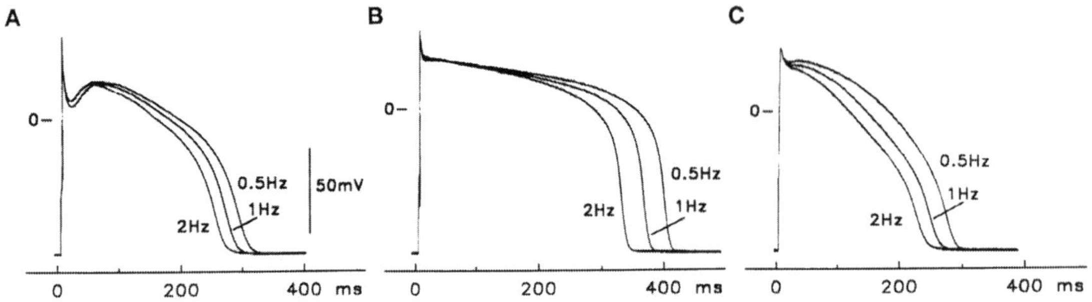

Figure 2.5: *Action potential curves measured on myocytes isolated from subepicardial (A), midmyocardial (B) and subendocardial (C) layers of the right ventricle of a human heart [5]. The curves were measured for different excitation frequencies (0.5, 1 and 2 Hz).*

right ventricle is 88% of its value in the left ventricle whereas only marginal difference has been detected for endocardium [31].

A method for estimation of the myocardial APD dispersion was described in [32, 33]. The inverse problem of electrocardiography is solved in order to reconstruct the isochrons of de- and repolarization fronts on the surface of the heart. This approach is based on an equivalent surface source model introduced in [34]. Under the assumption, that the conductivity anisotropy ratio in intra- and in extracellular space of the myocardium are equal, the ECG is fully defined by the excitation and relaxation of the cardiac surface. On the contrary, this equality is not confirmed by measurements [35]. It is shown by the author of this thesis in [36], that the unequal anisotropy ratio of conductivity in intra- and extracellular spaces of the bidomain enables the M-cells to contribute to the form of the ECG. Thus the method of inverse problem solution based on the equivalent surface sources needs to be validated both theoretically and clinically.

2.4 Cardiac Diseases: Infarction and Heart Blocks

2.4.1 Myocardial Infarction

A plug in a coronary artery or one of its branches supplying the ventricular myocardium with blood results in myocardial infarction (MI) [15]. MI in the right ventricle or in the atria are extremely seldom. As a result of this plug, the ventricular myocardium will show a deficiency of oxygen. The acidification of myocardial tissue with the end products of metabolism, which cannot be carried away by the blood, results in ischemia. The myocardium in the affected area looses its ability to contract, an infarction scar appears (see figure 2.6).

Myocardial infarctions are subdivided into two major categories. Transmural infarctions affect the whole depth of myocardium. The QRS-complex changes its shape strongly. Due to the pathological shape of the Q-wave, this type of infarction is often called *Q-wave infarction*.

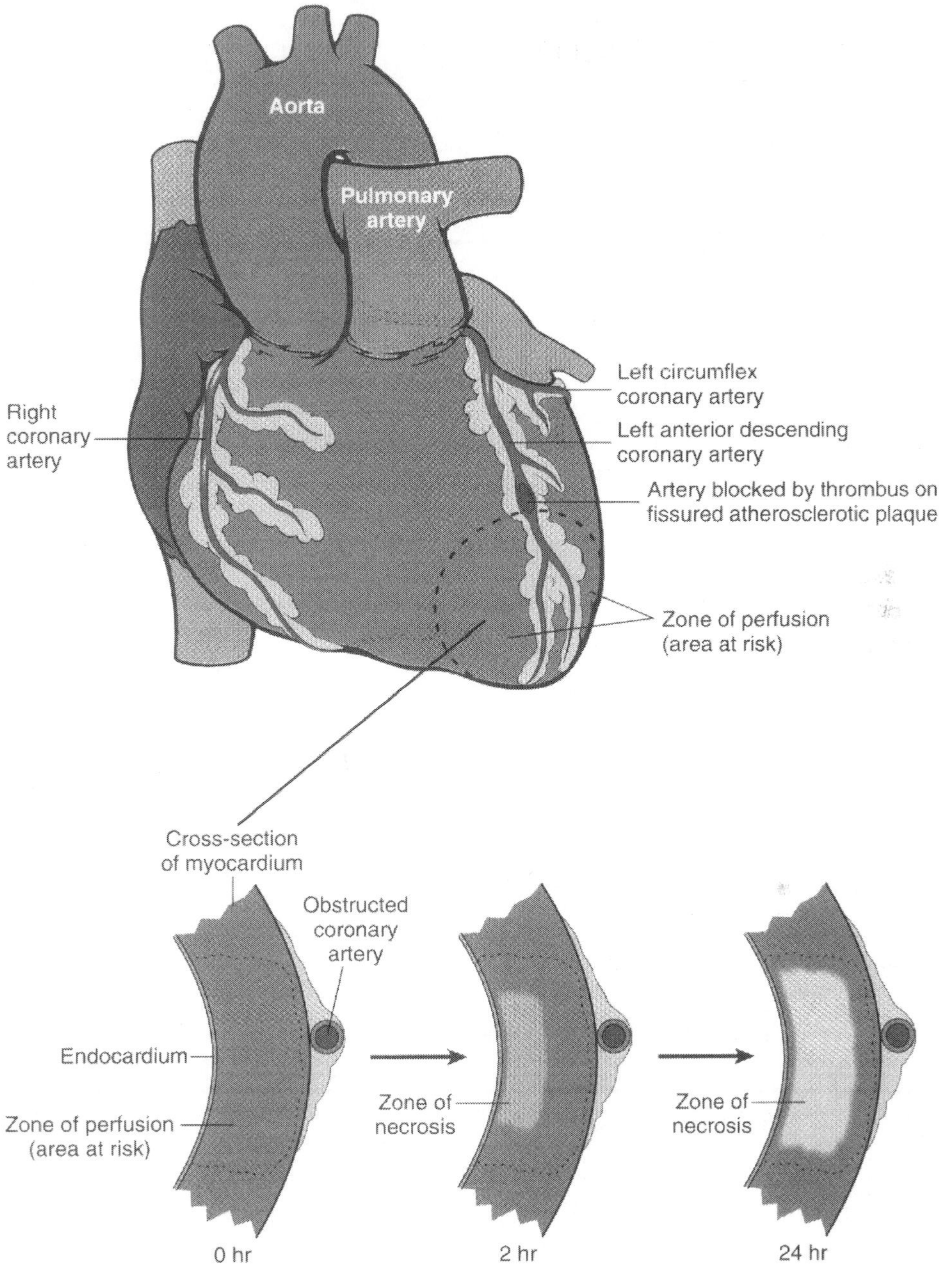

Figure 2.6: *Development of an infarction scar. The upper figure shows the site of possible infarction scar due to the closure of a coronary artery. The bottom figures show the development of necrotic tissue with the time [6].*

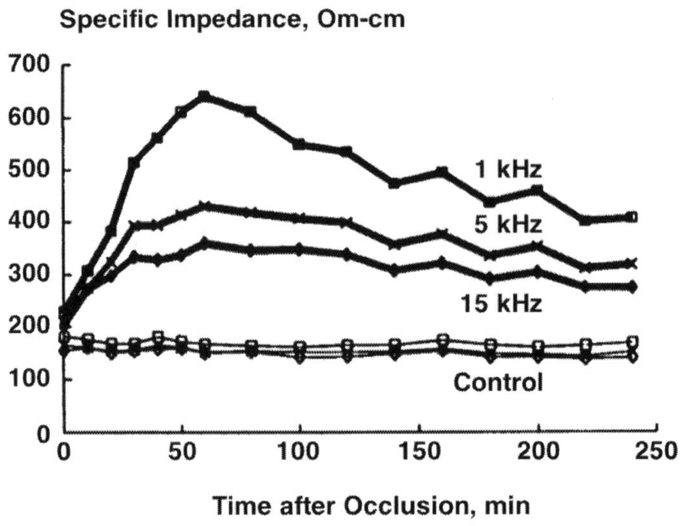

Figure 2.7: *Time course of the specific impedance of infarcted myocardium measured at 1, 5 and 15 kHz during the first 4 hours after coronary occlusion [7].*

Non-Q-wave infarctions do not normally expand to the whole depth of myocardium and thus cause only minor changes to the shape of the QRS-complex. Such infarctions can be diagnosed by the changes in ST-segment and in the T-wave. This kind of infarction can be subdivided into subendocardial and subepicardial.

A change of extracellular conductivity in ischemic as well as infarcted myocardium was reported in [7]. An artificial infarction was introduced by a ligation of a coronary artery in a sheep, afterwards the change of the specific impedance of affected myocardial tissue with time was registered. According to these measurements, the specific impedance of the ventricular tissue was increasing during the first 60 minutes after coronary occlusion by 200%, afterwards it started decreasing, ending up at 56% of that in non-infarcted region by the end of the 2nd week. The time course of the average specific impedance of infarcted myocardium during the first 240 minutes after coronary occlusion is shown in figure 2.7.

2.4.2 Bundle Branch Blocks

Due to various pathologies different branches of the excitation conduction system can be blocked. If the block is located right after the AV-node, the excitation cannot reach the ventricles, thus the cardiac contraction is completely disabled. Another possibility is a block of the left or right Tawara bundles, which is called left and right bundle branch block, correspondingly (see figure 2.8).

In the case of a right bundle branch block, the left ventricle is excited first, afterwards the excitation has to pass the septum in order to reach the right ventricle. Normal physiological excitation of the right ventricle is disabled. Such pathology leads to dyssynchrony of the cardiac contraction, which furthermore results in the decrease of ejection fraction

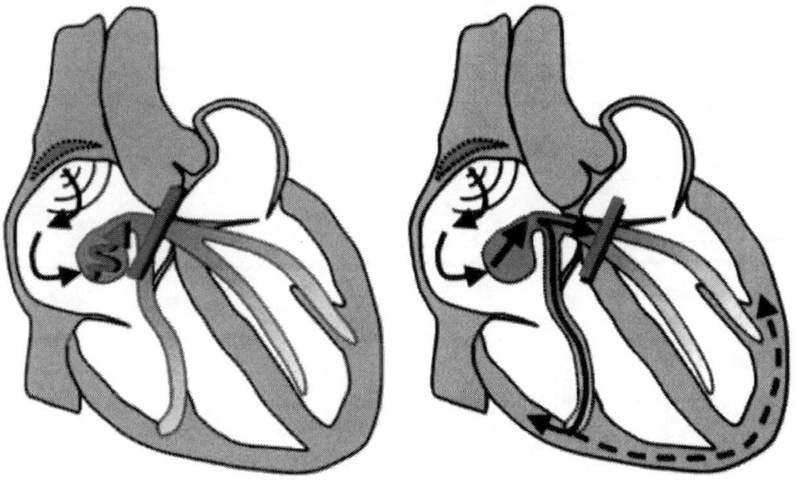

Figure 2.8: *Atrio-ventricular bundle branch block (left) and left bundle branch block (right). In the first case excitation does not reach the ventricles. In the second case the left ventricle is excited only through the right ventricular excitation [8].*

and arterial pressure [37].

Correspondingly, left bundle branch block results in the pathological excitation sequence of the left ventricle, which also decreases the ejection fraction.

The bundle branch blocks can be complete, fully isolating a part of excitation conduction system from the pacing tissue, and incomplete, introducing a significant delay into excitation propagation.

The ECG of a patient with a bundle branch block is characterized by a QRS-complex with the duration of more than 0.12 s and complicated form due to the asynchronous depolarization of the ventricles [38].

Chapter 3

Cardiac Modeling

3.1 Modeling the Anatomy of the Heart

The anatomical model of the heart is created using MRI or CT data sets. In the course of segmentation the tissues are classified and their borders are determined. A typical result of segmentation is shown in figure 3.1. A tissue class index is assigned to each significant organ afterwards, corresponding to a single record in the list of electrical and mechanical properties of the tissue.

Several segmentation methods were implemented at the Institute of Biomedical Engineering, Universität Karlsruhe (TH) originally in order to perform the segmentation of Visible Man [39] and Visible Female [40, 41] data sets. These methods are considered in this section.

Region Growing

Region growing is one of the most simple ways to extract a single organ out of the MRI data set. It is based on the fact that the voxels corresponding to the same organ possess (approximately) the same gray scale values and are interconnected. Thus one can select a range of interest, to which the gray scale values of the needed organ belong. Then a seed point within the organ is selected by the user. The algorithm checks, if the gray value of this voxel is within the range. If the voxel fits, a region of selection is created. Then all the neighboring voxels of the region are checked recursively, expanding the selection to the voxels which fit into the range. The process ends when all the neighboring voxels of the selected region have the gray values outside the range of interest [42].

In order to reduce the pixel noise of the MRI scans, median filtering was applied before segmentation.

The benefits of this segmentation method are relative simpleness of implementation and high level of automaticity. To its disadvantages belongs the instability of the method: if the organ being segmented has a neighboring organ with similar gray values, both organs will be selected together. If the organ of interest has two neighbors, one of them being "brighter" and the other "darker", then the voxels belonging to the border zone between

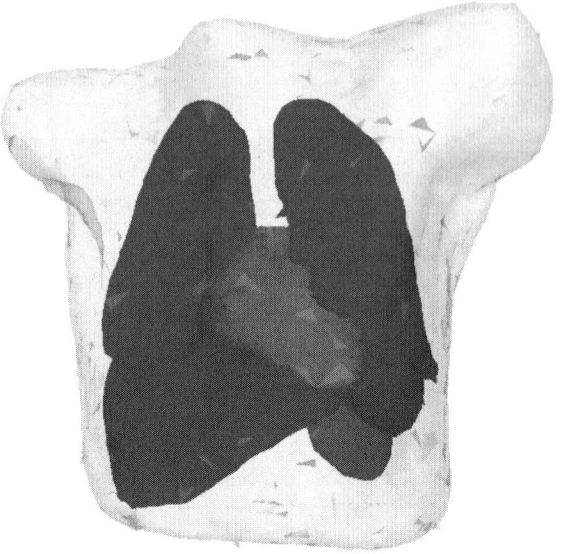

Figure 3.1: *Anatomical model of the patient's thorax resulting from the segmentation of an MRI data set. Lungs, heart, liver, spleen and kidneys are shown. The segmentation was performed using the deformable triangle meshes technique (see section 3.1).*

them can also have the same gray values, so the algorithm will also select them.

Deformable Triangle Meshes

Another method to perform the segmentation of a data set is to create triangle meshes reproducing the borders of the organs. There are two approaches, manual and automatic segmentation. In both cases an original mesh of a primitive form is created, normally a sphere, cylinder or plane. Then, in the course of manual segmentation, the user pushes and pulls different parts of the mesh in order to fit it to the borders of the segmented organ. The radial-basis-function-transformation is applied in order to perform a smooth deformation of the mesh in 3-dimensional space [43, 44]. The neighborhood relations in the surface mesh are taken into account.

Automatic segmentation is usually performed using so called "snakes" in 2D and triangle meshes representing "balloons" in 3D. The segmentation process consists in the minimization of a user-defined energy term by the deformation of the contour, until the best possible correspondence between the contour and the surface of the segmented organ is achieved. Several approaches were implemented and extended at the Institute of Biomedical Engineering, Universität Karlsruhe (TH), including "active contours" [45, 46] and "active shape models" [47, 48, 49].

3.2 Classification of Electrophysiological Cardiac Models

There exist several approaches to create a model of cardiac electrophysiology. Basically they can be subdivided into two main categories: mono- and bidomain modeling as well as rule-based modeling. The former considers the heart to consist of two subspaces, extra- and intracellular, being separated with the cell membrane. The membrane contains ion channels which allow ions of certain types to pass through it. The conductivity of ion channels changes according to the potential difference between the subspaces (transmembrane voltage – TMV). Thus a large amount of differential equations must be solved in order to simulate electrophysiology of myocardium. This task requires huge computational efforts, strong parallelization and large volumes of memory, but leads to very precise results.

Rule-based modeling, on the other hand, considers the excitation of small patches of ventricular tissue based on certain rules ignoring the nature of this excitation. These patches possess relatively large size (typically $1 \times 1 \times 1mm^3$), thus the memory consumption is moderate. The action potential curve, refractory times and excitation conduction velocity are not computed in the course of modeling, but selected from a database according to certain criteria. Thus the calculation time decreases dramatically (several minutes against several days for the bidomain models on a single workstation), which allows for the use of cardiac modeling in everyday clinical practice. Due to the relative simplicity of this approach, several cardiac models based on this principle have been developed [50, 51, 52, 53, 54, 55].

Both approaches have been implemented at the Institute of Biomedical Engineering, University of Karlsruhe (TH). In this work, bidomain models were used to generate the rules, which were afterwards employed by the rule-based cardiac model. In the following sections this collaboration is discussed in more detail.

Lately a hybrid between these two approaches is gaining relevance. A significantly simplified cell model like e.g. FitzHugh-Nagumo [56] coupled with a monodomain model can also lead to realistic results within a short time. Such approach would be especially effective for the modeling of arrhythmias.

3.3 General Scheme of Myocardial Cell Models

The first quantitative model of an excitable cell was proposed by Hodgkin and Huxley in [9]. They considered the cell membrane as an electrical circuit containing a capacity and three resistances plugged in parallel (see figure 3.2). The resistances were defined for the currents of sodium and potassium ions flowing through the corresponding ion channels, as well as for a small "leakage current" made up by chloride and other ions. The resistance for the latter current was considered to be constant, whereas the former two resistances were changing with the transmembrane voltage.

The total current through the cell membrane can be written as

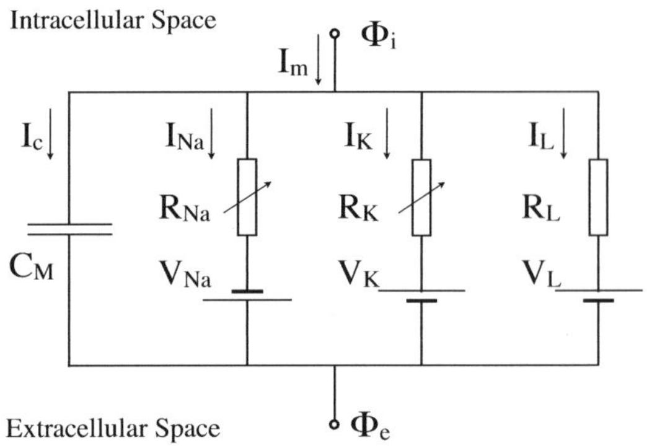

Figure 3.2: *The Hodgkin-Huxley representation of the cell membrane. Here I_m represents the transmembrane current, Φ_i and Φ_e are the intra- and extracellular potentials, with transmembrane voltage: $V_m = \Phi_i - \Phi_e$. I_{Na}, I_K and I_L represent the sodium, potassium and leakage currents, R_{Na}, R_K and R_L – corresponding resistances and V_{Na}, V_K and V_L - corresponding Nernst potentials. C_M is the capacitance of the cell membrane.*

$$I = C_M \cdot \frac{dV_m}{dt} + I_{Na} + I_K + I_L, \tag{3.1}$$

where I is the overall current through the cell membrane, C_M is the capacitance of the cell membrane, V_m is the transmembrane voltage (TMV), I_{Na}, I_K and I_L represent the sodium, potassium and leakage currents, correspondingly.

The ionic currents through the membrane can be computed by

$$I_{Na} = g_{Na} \cdot (V_m - V_{Na}), \tag{3.2}$$

$$I_K = g_K \cdot (V_m - V_K), \tag{3.3}$$

$$I_L = g_L \cdot (V_m - V_L), \tag{3.4}$$

where V_{Na}, V_K and V_L are the Nernst potentials for sodium, potassium and "leakage" ions [12], which are defined by the difference of concentration of the ion types inside and outside the cell, and g_{Na}, g_K and g_L are the corresponding conductivities. The latter are defined by the fraction of opened channels for each type of ions. They change according to first order differential equations. The rate constants of these differential equations depend on the TMV.

This model is able to correctly describe the excitation of an axon. The response of the cell to external excitations of different amplitudes (below or above the threshold) is shown in figure 3.3. Modern cell models reported in the literature are listed in table 3.1. They are specific for different types of excitable cells and different species (animals or human) and take into account much more types of ion channels in the membrane. All these cell models

Year	Author	Specimen	Species
1962	Noble [60]	Purkinje fiber	-
1975	McAllister, Noble, Tsien [61]	Purkinje fiber	-
1977	Beeler, Reuter [62]	Ventricular myocardium	Mammalian
1980	Yanagihara, Noma, Irisawa [63]	Sinoatrial node	Rabbit
1982	Bristow, Clark [64]	Sinoatrial node	Rabbit
1983	Bristow, Clark [65]	Sinoatrial node	Rabbit
1984	Noble, Noble [66]	Sinoatrial node	Rabbit
1985	DiFrancesco, Noble [67]	Purkinje fiber	Mammalian
1987	Hilgemann, Noble [68]	Atrial working myocardium	Rabbit
1990	Earm, Noble [69]	Atrial working myocardium	Rabbit
1991	Luo, Rudy [70]	Ventricular myocardium	Mammalian
1994	Luo, Rudy [71, 72]	Ventricular myocardium	Guinea-pig
1994	Demir, Clark, Murphey, Giles [73]	Sinoatrial node	Rabbit
1996	Dokos, Celler, Lovell [74]	Sinoatrial node	Mammalian
1996	Lindblad, Murphey, Clark, Giles [75]	Atrial working myocardium	Rabbit
1996	Demir, O'Rourke, Tomaselli, Marban, Winslow [76]	Ventricular myocardium	Rabbit
1998	Courtemanche, Ramirez, Nattel [77]	Atrial working myocardium	Human
1998	Nygren, Fiset, Firek, Clark, Lindblad, Clark, Giles [78]	Atrial working myocardium	Human
1998	Jafri, Rice, Winslow [79]	Ventricular myocardium	Guinea-pig
1998	Noble, Varghese, Kohl, Noble [80]	Ventricular myocardium	Guinea-pig
1998	Priebe, Beuckelmann [81]	Ventricular myocardium	Human
1999	Demir, Clark, Giles [82]	Sinoatrial node	Rabbit
1999	Winslow, Rice, Jafri, Marbán, O'Rourke [83]	Ventricular myocardium	Canine
2000	Ramirez, Nattel, Courtemanche [84]	Atrial working myocardium	Canine
2000	Zhang, Holden, Kodoma, Honjo, Lei, Varghese, Boyett [85]	Sinoatrial node	Rabbit
2001	Boyett, Zhang, Garny, Holden [86]	Sinoatrial node	Rabbit
2001	Pandit, Clark, Giles, Demir [87]	Ventricular myocardium	Rat
2001	Puglisi, Bers [88]	Ventricular myocardium	Rabbit
2002	Kneller, Ramirez, Chartier, Courtemanche, Nattel [89]	Atrial working myocardium	Canine
2002	Kurata, Hisatome, Imanishi, Shibamoto [90]	Sinoatrial node	Rabbit
2002	Bernus, Wilders, Zemlin, Verschelde, Panfilov [91]	Ventricular myocardium	Human
2004	Lovell, Cloherty, Celler, Dokos [92]	Sinoatrial node	Rabbit
2004	Ten Tusscher, Noble, Noble, Panfilov [22]	Ventricular myocardium	Human
2004	Iyer, Mazhari, Winslow [93]	Ventricular myocardium	Human

Table 3.1: *Cell models describing different cardiac tissues for different species [58]*

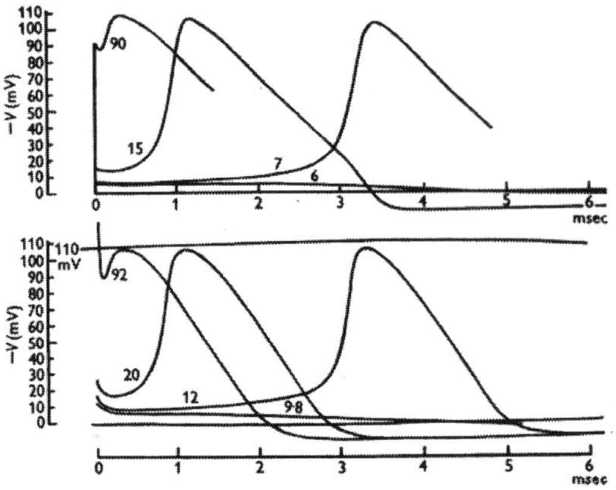

Figure 3.3: *Upper curves: solutions of eq. 3.1 for initial depolarizations of 90, 15, 7 and 6 mV (calculated for 6°C). Lower curves: tracings of membrane action potentials recorded at 6°C from an axon [9].*

have been implemented at the Institute of Biomedical Engineering, Universität Karlsruhe (TH) [57, 58, 59].

Another important factor taken into account by recently published bidomain models is the transmural dispersion of action potential duration [22, 23]. Research is currently performed to implement also the apico-basal and interventricular dispersions of the membrane properties.

3.4 Cellular Automaton

A cellular automaton based model of the heart used in the present work belongs to the rule-based heart models. This model does not consider the interaction between the intra- and extracellular spaces in order to simulate the excitation propagation. Instead, a set of rules is defined for this propagation. The action potential curves are not computed "on-the-fly", but rather chosen from a predefined library. Thus a high performance and low memory consumption are assured, although the method is by far not as flexible as the bidomain methods.

A cellular automaton is applied to simulate the excitation propagation throughout the heart. If a voxel is depolarized, under certain conditions the neighboring voxels get excited as well. A voxel is considered as neighboring to a given one, if they have a common face or if they are connected with a segment of the excitation conduction system.

The excitation is conducted between the voxels if the following conditions are met:

1. Both voxels are excitable.

2. Both voxels belong to the same tissue or to tissues, between which the excitation conduction is allowed. For example, the direct conduction of excitation from atria to

ventricles and vice versa is forbidden. On the contrary, the excitation propagation between Purkinje fibers and ventricular myocardium is allowed.

3. The voxel receiving the excitation should not be already excited. In other words, the myocardial tissue within the voxel should not be in refractory state.

For a normal heart beat, the excitation starts in the AV-node with a given frequency defining the heart rate. Afterwards the excitation propagates through the excitation conduction system and reaches the ventricular myocardium. There the excitation propagation continues according to conditions described in section 3.5. The TMV distributions corresponding to a normal heart beat are shown in figure 7.8.

An extrasystolic beat can be modeled by introduction of a spontaneous excitation somewhere in the myocardium. Then the excitation is conducted through the myocardium until it reaches the excitation conduction system. Afterwards the excitation is spread over the endocardium by the conduction system. So the "all-or-nothing" principle (see chapter 2) is fulfilled independently from the origin of excitation. The TMV distributions for an extrasystolic heart beat are shown in figure 7.10.

The cellular automaton computes the distributions of TMV with the step of 0.1 ms, after each 4 ms the TMV distribution is saved on disk.

3.5 Electrophysiological Properties of Myocardial Tissue

The voxels of the anatomical heart model described in section 7.1 are characterized by several values defining their electrophysiological properties and excitation behavior. These values are listed and characterized in this section.

3.5.1 Tissue Class

The main property of each voxel is its tissue class. This is an integer value between 0 and 255, which is used as a key in several tables defining

- the electrical conductivity and magnetic permeability of the voxel;
- its mechanical properties;
- its response to external stimulation.

The electrical conductivity of each tissue class was taken from the literature [35, 94]. The relative magnetic permeability was assumed to be 1 for all tissue classes. Excitable tissues are characterized by their extra- and intracellular conductivities σ_e and σ_i; these values are used to solve the bidomain equations (see chapter 4).

The response of a voxel to external stimuli is described by the following characteristics:

1. The excitability of the tissue;
2. A set of action potential curves corresponding to different stimulation frequencies as well as to different refractory states of the voxel;
3. Excitation conduction velocity (isotropic and/or anisotropic) and refractory times for different stimulation frequencies and refractory states;
4. A list of tissues, to which the excitation is allowed to be conducted;
5. Automaticity determining the frequency of autostimulation.

The voxels that are not excitable are ignored by the model and do not contribute to the generation of ECG. It should be noted although, that "excitable" voxels might also be unable to depolarize (see section 7.4).

3.5.2 Other Characteristics

A float value between 0 and 1 defines the location of the voxel within the ventricle wall, with 0 corresponding to the endocardial and 1 to the epicardial surface. This value is defined only for the ventricular myocardium. It is used to emulate the transmural dispersion of action potentials. A set of 97 action potentials for different layers is created (see section 7.3). An additional application of this information is to modify the infarction area (see section 7.4).

Another float value is used to modify the behavior of ventricular myocardium neighboring to the area of myocardial infarction. It contains the factor by which the amplitude of action potential, excitation conduction velocity and action potential duration in the given voxel is multiplied. The modeling of infarction is described in Section 7.4 in more detail.

Chapter 4

Forward Problem of Electrocardiography

4.1 Formulation of the Forward Problem

The forward problem of electrocardiography consists in the computation of the body surface potential map (BSPM) corresponding to a given distribution of transmembrane voltages within the heart. The main applications of the forward problem are:

- Investigation of the influence of electrophysiological properties (such as geometry, conductivity, anisotropy etc) of various tissues on the resulting ECG;
- Validation of the results obtained from the electrophysiological heart models (see Chapter 3);
- Optimization of the ECG measurements (e.g. electrode locations);
- Computation of the transfer matrix for the inverse problem of electrocardiography.

The Poisson equation describes the relation between the impressed current sources within the myocardium and the potential distributions within the volume conductor representing the patient's torso. As the ECG of the patient does not contain frequencies exceeding 1 kHz, the impedance of the torso is to an excellent approximation just resistive, and the phase shift of the bioelectrical field on its way from the heart to the body surface is negligible. Thus the problem is quasi-stationary. This means, that the distribution of potentials within the torso at a given time instant depends only on the distribution of cardiac sources at the very time instant. Furthermore, the problem is linear, which means that the potentials caused by a set of cardiac sources is equal to the sum of potentials caused by each of these sources [34].

In the present work the transmembrane voltages obtained from the cellular automaton heart model were interpolated on the tetrahedron mesh of the volume conductor representing the anatomical torso model. Afterwards the bidomain approach was employed to compute the distribution of the extracellular potentials within the thorax.

As the human thorax has a complicated geometry, it is quite difficult to perform the computations directly. There are two possible ways around this problem. First, the geometry can be reduced to some primitive shape (like in the eccentric spheres model [95]). Another approach is to discretize the geometry into homogeneous subdomains and employ the computational methods to solve the problem.

In this work, the finite element method [96] is utilized. The volume conductor is subdivided into tetrahedral elements each containing some homogeneous tissue. The size of the elements can be varied in different subdomains of the solution domain, with the average size of 2 mm within the ventricular myocardium and of circa 10 mm within the lungs. Thus an efficient memory consumption and a reduced computation time are assured.

The main complication of this approach consists in the generation of high-quality unstructured tetrahedral grids which is by itself an important area of research [97].

4.2 Bidomain Model

The bidomain model is a macroscopic way to consider the cellular electrophysiology of the cardiac tissue. The myocardial region is subdivided into spatially coinciding intra- and extracellular subspaces, each possessing its own potential distribution and conductivity tensor. These values are described by the following system of equations:

$$\nabla \cdot (\sigma_i \nabla \varphi_i) = \beta I_m, \tag{4.1}$$

$$\nabla \cdot (\sigma_e \nabla \varphi_e) = -\beta I_m, \tag{4.2}$$

where σ_i and φ_i are the conductivity tensor and the potential in the intracellular space, σ_e and φ_e correspond to the extracellular space and β is the membrane surface-to-volume ratio. The conductivity tensors σ_e and σ_i for the anisotropical tissues (e.g. ventricular myocardium) are defined in the coordinate system based on the fiber orientation as:

$$\sigma_e = \begin{pmatrix} \sigma_{e,l} & 0 & 0 \\ 0 & \sigma_{e,t} & 0 \\ 0 & 0 & \sigma_{e,t} \end{pmatrix} \tag{4.3}$$

and

$$\sigma_i = \begin{pmatrix} \sigma_{i,l} & 0 & 0 \\ 0 & \sigma_{i,t} & 0 \\ 0 & 0 & \sigma_{i,t} \end{pmatrix}. \tag{4.4}$$

Here $\sigma_{e,l}$ and $\sigma_{i,l}$ denote the extra- and intracellular conductivities along the fiber direction (longitudinal), whereas $\sigma_{e,t}$ and $\sigma_{i,t}$ represent the corresponding conductivities perpendicular to this direction (transversal). The ratio between longitudinal and transversal conductivities in each subspace is called *anisotropy ratio* in that subspace.

The transmembrane current density I_m consists of a capacitive part (displacement current), the ionic currents and the imposed stimulation current [98].

Adding equations (4.1) and (4.2) and considering $\varphi_i = \varphi_e + V_m$, where V_m is the transmembrane voltage, we obtain the dependency between the extracellular potential and the transmembrane voltage:

$$\nabla \cdot ((\sigma_i + \sigma_e)\nabla\varphi_e) = -\nabla \cdot (\sigma_i \nabla V_m). \tag{4.5}$$

The bidomain area can be extended to the whole volume conductor, with $\sigma_i = 0$ for the region outside of the active tissue. Thus we guarantee that φ_e is continuous across the boundary of the myocardium, and the normal component of the intracellular current vanishes on this boundary.

If the overall conductivity of the bidomain $(\sigma_i + \sigma_e)$ is replaced with σ, the extracellular potential φ_e with φ and the impressed current source density $\nabla \cdot (\sigma_i \nabla V_m)$ with f, then the Poisson's equation is obtained:

$$\nabla \cdot (\sigma \nabla \varphi) = -f \text{ in } \Omega, \tag{4.6}$$

where Ω is a finite domain of the volume conductor. Its boundary Γ consists of two parts: Γ_1, where the zero reference potential is defined (Dirichlet boundary condition), and Γ_2, the boundary between the thorax and the air, where Neumann boundary conditions are applied:

$$\varphi = \varphi_D \text{ on } \Gamma_1, \tag{4.7}$$

$$(\sigma \nabla \varphi) \cdot \mathbf{n} = 0 \text{ on } \Gamma_2. \tag{4.8}$$

The problem (4.6-4.8) can be written in the variational form: find a function φ such that the functional

$$I(\varphi) = \frac{1}{2} \int\limits_{\Omega} [(\sigma \nabla \varphi) \cdot \nabla \varphi - 2f\varphi] \, dv \tag{4.9}$$

is stationary, and the Dirichlet boundary conditions (4.7) are satisfied.

The Rayleigh-Ritz method can be used to solve this variational problem. The method consists in the expansion of a function $\varphi(x, y, z)$ as a linear combination of basis functions $\psi_0, \psi_1, \psi_2, ..., \psi_n$. These functions should be linearly independent and form the full system on the region where the functional (4.9) is defined [99].

The function ψ_0 is chosen to satisfy the Dirichlet boundary conditions on Γ_1, whereas the rest of the basis functions are chosen to be zero on Γ_1 [11]. Thus the approximate solution of the problem (4.9, 4.7) can be written as

$$\tilde{\varphi} = \psi_0 + \sum_{i=1}^{n} a_i \psi_i. \tag{4.10}$$

Substituting (4.10) into (4.9), we obtain the functional $I(\varphi)$ depending only on the unknown coefficients a_i, with $i = 1..n$. This functional is stationary if the following conditions are satisfied:

$$\frac{\partial I}{\partial a_i} = 0, i = 1, 2, ..., n. \tag{4.11}$$

With this respect, a system of n linear equations can be built in order to find the unknown coefficients a_i:

$$\begin{gathered}\sum_{j=1}^{n}\left(\int_{\Omega}(\sigma\nabla\psi_i)\nabla\psi_j dv\right)a_j + \int_{\Omega}[(\sigma\nabla\psi_i)\nabla\psi_0 - f\psi_i]dv = 0,\\ i = 1, 2, ..., n.\end{gathered} \tag{4.12}$$

By solving this system the coefficients a_i for the solution (4.10) can be found. The Dirichlet boundary conditions are satisfied due to the choice of functions ψ_i, and the Neumann boundary conditions are satisfied as they are included into the formulation (4.9).

4.3 Discretization of the Solution Domain

As it was mentioned in section 4.1, a tetrahedral unstructured grid is created upon which the forward (and inverse, see Chapter 5) calculations are performed. For each tetrahedron 4 linear *element shape functions* $N_i^{(e)}$ are defined, one for each node. These functions have the value 1 on the corresponding node, and 0 at the other nodes of the tetrahedron [96]:

$$N_i^{(e)} = \begin{cases} 1, & i = j \\ 0, & i \neq j. \end{cases} \tag{4.13}$$

Another important property of the functions $N_i^{(e)}$ is the following: the sum of these functions is equal to 1 at each point of the tetrahedron:

$$\sum_{i=1}^{4} N_i^{(e)}(\vec{r}) = 1 \;\forall\, \vec{r} \in \Omega^{(e)}, \tag{4.14}$$

where $\Omega^{(e)}$ is the space occupied by the tetrahedron.

Let's now consider a single node of the mesh. It builds up several tetrahedra. If we sum up the element shape functions of this node in all these tetrahedra, we obtain a linear *node shape function* N_k for this node (see figure 4.1), where k is the index of the node, $k = 1..n$, with n being the number of nodes in the grid.

Thus, the distribution of potentials within the volume conductor can be approximately represented by

$$\tilde{\varphi} = \sum_{k=1}^{n} \varphi_k N_k, \tag{4.15}$$

where φ_k is the electrical potential on the node k. As the node shape functions N_k are linearly independent, and comprise the full set of functions in the domain Ω, functions ψ_k in the equation (4.12) can be replaced by N_k:

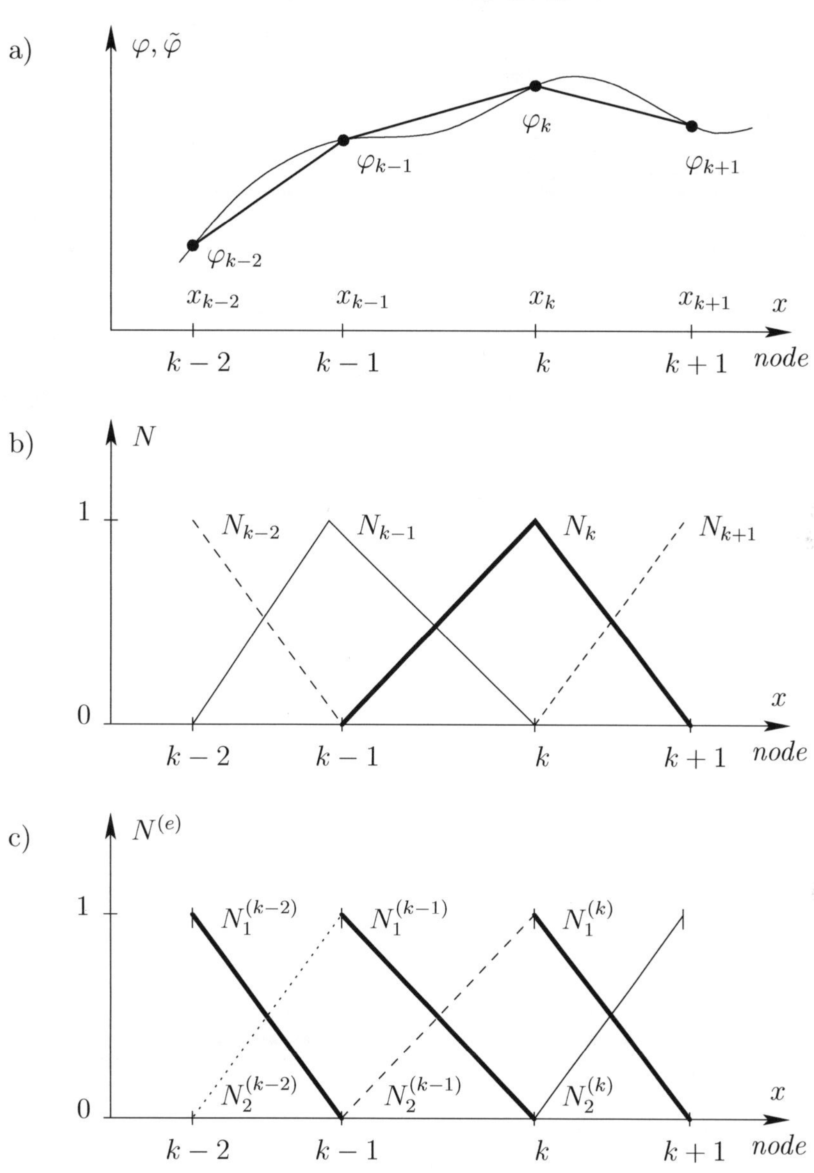

Figure 4.1: *Finite element approximation of a function φ in a one-dimensional domain (a). Node interpolation functions N_k serve as a basis for the approximation (b). They are constructed as a superposition of the element interpolation functions (c) [11].*

$$\sum_{j=1}^{n}\left(\int_{\Omega}(\sigma\nabla N_i)\nabla N_j dv\right)\varphi_j - \int_{\Omega} f N_i dv = 0,\ i = 1, 2, ..., n. \tag{4.16}$$

Considering the integrals $\int_{\Omega}(\sigma\nabla N_i)\nabla N_j dv$ as the elements of the *system matrix* $S \in \mathbb{R}^{n\times n}$, and $\int_{\Omega} f N_i dv$ as the elements of the vector of sources $\vec{b} \in \mathbb{R}^n$, the equation 4.16 can be reduced to the form

$$S\vec{\varphi} = \vec{b}. \tag{4.17}$$

The computation of the elements of S and $\vec{b}$ is described in [96, 11]. The system matrix here is sparse, because ∇N_i is 0 at all nodes except the i-th one and its neighbors. It is also positive definite, which means that $\xi^T \cdot S\xi > 0\ \forall\ \xi \in \mathbb{R}^n$. And, finally, the matrix is symmetric.

4.3.1 Handling the Dirichlet Boundary Conditions

Equation (4.17) can be reduced by taking the Dirichlet boundary conditions into account. Let $\varphi_k = \Phi_k$ be the Dirichlet boundary condition set at the node k. This condition can be included into the equation (4.17) by setting the element s_{kk} of the matrix S to 1, the rest of the elements in the kth row to 0, and b_k to Φ_k:

$$\begin{pmatrix} s_{11} & s_{12} & \dots & s_{1k} & \dots & s_{1n} \\ s_{21} & s_{22} & \dots & s_{2k} & \dots & s_{2n} \\ \vdots & \vdots & \ddots & \vdots & & \vdots \\ 0 & 0 & \dots & 1 & \dots & 0 \\ \vdots & \vdots & & \vdots & \ddots & \vdots \\ s_{n1} & s_{n2} & \dots & s_{nk} & \dots & s_{nn} \end{pmatrix} \begin{pmatrix} \varphi_1 \\ \varphi_2 \\ \vdots \\ \varphi_k \\ \vdots \\ \varphi_n \end{pmatrix} = \begin{pmatrix} b_1 \\ b_2 \\ \vdots \\ \Phi_k \\ \vdots \\ b_n \end{pmatrix}. \tag{4.18}$$

To preserve the symmetry of the system matrix, the none-diagonal elements of the kth column were also set to 0:

$$\begin{pmatrix} s_{11} & s_{12} & \dots & 0 & \dots & s_{1n} \\ s_{21} & s_{22} & \dots & 0 & \dots & s_{2n} \\ \vdots & \vdots & \ddots & \vdots & & \vdots \\ 0 & 0 & \dots & 1 & \dots & 0 \\ \vdots & \vdots & & \vdots & \ddots & \vdots \\ s_{n1} & s_{n2} & \dots & 0 & \dots & s_{nn} \end{pmatrix} \begin{pmatrix} \varphi_1 \\ \varphi_2 \\ \vdots \\ \varphi_k \\ \vdots \\ \varphi_n \end{pmatrix} = \begin{pmatrix} b_1 - s_{1k}\Phi_k \\ b_2 - s_{2k}\Phi_k \\ \vdots \\ \Phi_k \\ \vdots \\ b_n - s_{nk}\Phi_k \end{pmatrix}. \tag{4.19}$$

After the insertion of boundary conditions the system matrix remains positive definite [100].

4.3.2 Computation of the Source Term

The source term f in equation (4.16), representing the impressed current density, is usually unknown. Therefore the computation of this term from the given distributions of TMV is needed, with $f = \nabla \cdot (\sigma_i \nabla V_m)$. Let's get rid of misleading indices, replacing V_m with V and σ_i with $\tilde{\sigma}$. Then the source term in (4.16) can be computed as follows:

$$\mathcal{I} = \int\limits_{\Omega} \nabla \cdot (\tilde{\sigma} \nabla V)\, N_i dv. \tag{4.20}$$

According to the divergence theorem, equation (4.20) can be re-written as

$$\mathcal{I} = \oint\limits_{\Gamma} \nabla \cdot (\tilde{\sigma} \nabla V)\, N_i ds - \int\limits_{\Omega} \cdot (\tilde{\sigma} \nabla V)\, \nabla N_i dv. \tag{4.21}$$

As the intracellular conductivity $\tilde{\sigma} = 0$ outside of the myocardial tissue, and the transmembrane voltage is constant in the tissues surrounding the heart ($\nabla V = 0$), the integration domain can be extended on the whole volume conductor, and the first integral in (4.21) is obviously equal to zero:

$$\mathcal{I} = -\int\limits_{\Omega} \cdot (\tilde{\sigma} \nabla V)\, \nabla N_i dv. \tag{4.22}$$

The TMV V can be re-written in terms of node interpolation functions like in equation (4.15):

$$V = \sum_{j=1}^{n} V_j N_j. \tag{4.23}$$

Therefore, taking the symmetry of the conductivity tensor into account, (4.22) can be transformed to

$$\mathcal{I} = -\sum_{j=1}^{n} \left(\int\limits_{\Omega} (\tilde{\sigma} \nabla N_i)\, \nabla N_j dv \right) V_j. \tag{4.24}$$

Thus the computation of the source term $\vec{b}$ consists in the multiplication of the TMV values on the nodes of the mesh $\vec{V}$ with the matrix

$$\tilde{S}_{ij} = \int\limits_{\Omega} (\tilde{\sigma} \nabla N_i)\, \nabla N_j dv, \tag{4.25}$$

the elements of which are computed analogously to those of the system matrix in (4.16).

4.4 Solution of the Forward Problem

Previous sections described the transformation of Poisson's problem (4.6-4.8) to a system of linear equations of the form

$$S \cdot \vec{\varphi} = \vec{b}, \tag{4.26}$$

where $S \in \mathbb{R}^{n \times n}$ is the system matrix being sparse, symmetric and positive definite, $\vec{\varphi} \in \mathbb{R}^n$ is the vector of unknown potentials and $\vec{b} \in \mathbb{R}^n$ is the term denoting the impressed current density. There exist several methods to solve such systems.

4.4.1 Gaussian Elimination

The principle of Gaussian elimination consists in the transformation of matrix S in equation (4.26) to triangular form. This is done by using linear combinations of single equations.

For example, let us consider the following system of two equations:

$$\begin{array}{rcrcr} 3x_1 & + & 5x_2 & = & 12, \\ 9x_1 & + & 7x_2 & = & 8. \end{array}$$

If the first equation is multiplied by 3 and subtracted from the second one, the system can be reduced to the form

$$\begin{array}{rcrcr} 3x_1 & + & 5x_2 & = & 12 \\ & & -8x_2 & = & -28. \end{array}$$

In the matrix form this operation can be represented as the replacement of matrix S by a product of a lower triangular matrix L and upper triangular U:

$$S = L \cdot U,$$

which in this example results in

$$\begin{pmatrix} 3 & 5 \\ 9 & 7 \end{pmatrix} = \begin{pmatrix} 1 & 0 \\ 3 & 1 \end{pmatrix} \cdot \begin{pmatrix} 3 & 5 \\ 0 & -8 \end{pmatrix}.$$

This operation is called *LU-factorization*. If the matrices L and U are computed, the solution of the system of equations is trivial [100].

Let us assume that a diagonal matrix $D = diag(d_1, d_2, ..., d_n)$ is constructed with $d_i = u_{ii}$ and matrix M is computed such that $M^T = D^{-1}U$, then

$$S = LDM^T \tag{4.27}$$

and M is lower triangular with unit elements in the main diagonal. It can be shown that for symmetric matrices $M = L$ and $S = LDL^T$.

4.4.2 Cholesky Decomposition

It can be shown that for positive definite symmetric systems the values of d_i are positive. Then the matrix D can be replaced with a product of two equal diagonal matrices $D = \tilde{D} \cdot \tilde{D}$ with elements $\tilde{d}_i = \sqrt{d_i}$. In this case equation (4.27) can be transformed to

$$S = L\tilde{D}\tilde{D}L^T = YY^T, \tag{4.28}$$

where $Y = L\tilde{D}$. Matrix Y is obviously lower triangular. This factorization is called Cholesky decomposition.

If the nodes of the volume conductor model are renumbered properly, the nonzero elements of the system matrix can be grouped near the main diagonal, which improves the memory consumption and overall performance of the method.

4.4.3 Conjugate Gradient Method

The conjugate gradient (CG) method is an iterative method of solution of large linear systems. Its main advantage consists in much smaller memory consumption than that of the direct methods described above. Thus (well-defined) systems with virtually any number of unknowns can be solved.

Let us consider the following function:

$$f(\vec{x}) = \frac{1}{2}\vec{x}^T S \vec{x} - \vec{x}^T \vec{b}, \tag{4.29}$$

where S and $\vec{b}$ are the system matrix and the right-hand vector in equation (4.26) respectively. As S is positive definite and symmetric, the global minimum of function $f(\vec{x})$ is located in the point $\vec{x} = S^{-1}\vec{b}$ [100]. Thus the minimization of $f(\vec{x})$ is equivalent to the solution of equation (4.26) with $\vec{\varphi}$ replaced by $\vec{x}$.

Let us consider a vector space $\vec{p}_1, ..., \vec{p}_n$ denoting n independent search directions for optimization of $f(\vec{x})$. At each step k a quantity α_k must be found, for which $f(\vec{x}_{k-1} + \alpha_k \vec{p}_k)$ is minimal. Thus after n steps the global minimum of $f(\vec{x})$ is found and therefore equation (4.26) is solved.

The conjugate gradient method consists in the generation of the set of directions $\vec{p}_i$, $i = 1...n$, which are S-conjugate to each other:

$$\vec{p}_i^{\,T} A \vec{p}_j = 0, \quad i \neq j. \tag{4.30}$$

If $\vec{x}_0$ denotes the initial guess, the first vector of search direction $\vec{p}_1$ is found as

$$\vec{p}_1 = \vec{r}_0 = \vec{b} - A\vec{x}_0, \tag{4.31}$$

being the direction of steepest descent. The further iterations are performed as follows:

$$\vec{p}_k = \vec{r}_{k-1} + \beta_k \vec{p}_{k-1}, \quad \beta_k = \frac{\vec{r}_{k-1}^{\,T} \vec{r}_{k-1}}{\vec{r}_{k-2}^{\,T} \vec{r}_{k-2}}, \tag{4.32}$$

$$\vec{x}_k = \vec{x}_{k-1} + \alpha_k \vec{p}_k, \quad \alpha_k = \frac{\vec{r}_{k-1}^{\,T} \vec{r}_{k-1}}{\vec{p}_k^{\,T} A \vec{p}_k}, \tag{4.33}$$

$$\vec{r}_k = \vec{r}_{k-1} - \alpha_k A \vec{p}_k. \tag{4.34}$$

It can be shown that the residuals $\vec{r}_i$ are mutually orthogonal. Thus each iteration step eliminates a single component of residual, in the absence of numerical errors the residual should be 0 after exactly n steps. For large n the number of iterations needed to substantially decrease the residual is usually much smaller [11].

In the current work, Cholesky decomposition as well as conjugate gradient method with preconditioning [11, 100] are used in order to solve the problem (4.6-4.8). Thus if the distribution of transmembrane voltages is defined, the corresponding potential distribution within the patient's thorax can be computed.

Chapter 5

Inverse Problem of Electrocardiography

5.1 Formulation of the Inverse Problem

Inverse problems generally consider the reconstruction of the cause by its effects, as opposed to forward problems dealing with the prediction of effects for a known cause. The mathematical framework for this class of problems is nowadays used in many fields of science such as geophysics, optics, image processing and astronomy.

The most common feature of many inverse problems is their *ill-posedness*, which means, that the solution of this problem is not unique, and does not change continuously with the input data. This term was introduced by Hadamard in [101]. For the inverse problems this means that additional assumptions have to be introduced into the formulation of the problem in order to stabilize its solution (so-called *regularization* [102]).

In electrocardiography the methodology of inverse problems is used for imaging of the cardiac activity of a patient from multichannel ECG or MCG measurements [103, 104, 105, 106]. There exist several different approaches to represent the intracardiac sources and, correspondingly, to formulate the inverse problem.

5.1.1 Epi- and Endocardial Potentials

The task to reconstruct epi- and endocardial potentials is a classical equivalent source model. The first attempts to reconstruct the epicardial potentials from a measured BSPM date back to the seventies [107, 108]. The distribution of extracellular potentials on the surface of the ventricular myocardium is considered as the "sources". Epicardial potentials can be measured experimentally [109, 110], which enables a direct validation of reconstruction results (like, e.g., in [111, 112]). Another important area of application for this approach is the reconstruction of endocardial potentials given the results of catheter measurements [113, 114, 115]. The measurement of epi- and endocardial potentials is shown in figure 5.1 (a, b).

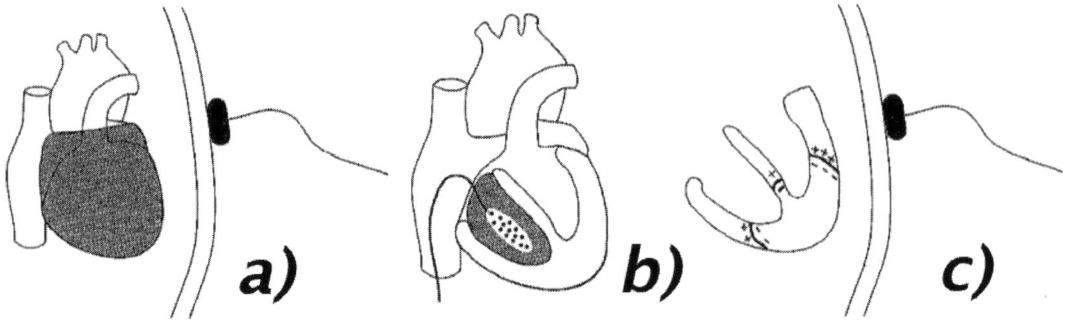

Figure 5.1: *Three formulations of the inverse problem of electrocardiography: epicardial potentials reconstructed from body surface potential mapping (a), endocardial potentials reconstructed from intracardiac catheter measurements (b), uniform double layer with activation times reconstructed from BSPM (c). Adopted from [10].*

An important trade-off of this equivalent source representation is the difficult interpretation of the reconstruction results: the potential in each point is defined by the distribution of TMV within the whole heart, not just from the sources in the neighborhood of that point.

In this work the term "epicardial potentials" will often be used with the meaning of "the distribution of potentials on the epi- and endocardial surfaces of the heart" for the sake of briefness.

5.1.2 Transmembrane Voltages

The bidomain model (see section 4.2) gives a linear relationship between the distributions of TMV within the myocardium and the BSPMs. Thus a linear inverse problem can be formulated in terms of TMV distributions as cardiac sources. A serious trade-off of this formulation consists in the non-uniqueness of its solution. Generally speaking, any distribution of TMV $V_m(\vec{r})$ which satisfies $\nabla \cdot (\sigma_i \nabla V_m) = 0$ results in zero ECG. This issue can be resolved by imposing additional constrains to the solution.

Still if the TMV distribution can be computed, it can fully define the state of the heart with high diagnostic value. Therefore this model of cardiac sources is used nowadays by several groups [116, 117, 118].

5.1.3 Uniform Double Layer

The uniform double layer of current dipoles (UDL) is another widely used representation of cardiac sources. It is assumed that the BSPM during the depolarization phase of the heart cycle is produced by a UDL lying along the activation front and oriented in its normal direction [10], like it is shown in figure 5.1 (*c*). Reconstructed is typically the time instance at which the UDL reaches the given point of the myocardium.

The basic equation of this approach is the following:

$$\int_{\Gamma_H} A(\vec{r}_B, \vec{r}_H) H(t - \tau(\vec{r}_H)) d\vec{r}_H = V(\vec{r}_B, t), \tag{5.1}$$

where $V(\vec{r}_B, t)$ is the body surface potential in point $\vec{r}_B$ at the time t, $A(\vec{r}_B, \vec{r}_H)$ represents the transfer function determined by the geometry of the thorax and the distribution of conductivities within it, $\tau(\vec{r}_H)$ is the activation time of the myocardium in point $\vec{r}_H$ of the heart surface Γ_H, and $H(t - \tau(\vec{r}_H))$ is the activation or deactivation function showing the dependence of TMV from time t at point $\vec{r}_H$, with activation or deactivation taking place at time $\tau(\vec{r}_H)$ [119]. The Heaviside step function is often employed to represent the change of TMV during the activation in each point of the heart.

The reconstruction of deactivation times from a measured sequence of BSPMs employing the UDL model is described in [32].

Thus the representation of the cardiac sources being reconstructed is not the TMV by itself, but rather the times when it changes.

From equation (5.1) it is clear, that the problem is basically non-linear. Within the scope of this approach only the surface of the heart is considered, which can lead to modeling errors due to the anisotropy of ventricular myocardium (see section 8.1, [36]).

An important advantage of this method is, on the other hand, the assumption of a "wavefront" behavior of the ventricular depolarization which employs an additional bias on the inverse problem, making it less ill-posed. Thus a more stable solution is to be expected.

A disadvantage is that the temporal slope of the function H has to be known beforehand for every position $\vec{r}_H$. Often for all positions the same function is applied which might be wrong in case of patients with ischemic or infarcted heart, although this significantly reduces the computation costs [120, 121].

Several clinical investigations employing this approach have been performed recently [122, 123], proving the stability and clinical reliability of the method.

In this work only the first two approaches (subsections 5.1.1 and 5.1.2) were implemented, the UDL model was left out of consideration.

5.2 Transfer Matrix

The linear relationship between the cardiac sources and the body surface potentials after the discretization of the solution domain can be written in matrix form:

$$A \cdot \vec{x} = \vec{y}, \tag{5.2}$$

where $A \in \mathbb{R}^{m \times n}$ is the transfer matrix describing the relationship between the cardiac sources and body surface potentials, with m being the number of electrodes and n representing the number of cardiac sources; $\vec{x} \in \mathbb{R}^n$ is the vector of unknown cardiac sources and $\vec{y} \in \mathbb{R}^m$ is the vector of measured BSPMs [11].

The computation of the transfer matrix A is an important – and rather time-consuming – part of the inverse problem. This matrix contains the information about the geometry and conductivity distribution of the volume conductor. Depending on the choice of equivalent cardiac sources, there exist different approaches to the computation of this matrix.

5.2.1 Transfer Matrix for Epi- and Endocardial Potentials

The transfer matrix expressing the dependence of BSPM on the distribution of epicardial potentials is also called *lead-field matrix*. Its computation consists in the reformulation of equation (4.17) with $\vec{b} = 0$ so that the potentials $\vec{\varphi}_H$ on the heart surface would be related to those measured on the electrodes $\vec{\varphi}_E$.

Let us subdivide the nodes of the finite element mesh on the subsets including a) nodes on the epi- and endocardium where the potentials are sought, b) electrode nodes where the BSPM is measured and c) all the rest of the nodes. The corresponding potentials will be defined as $\vec{\varphi}_H$, $\vec{\varphi}_E$ and $\vec{\varphi}_R$. Then the expression (4.17) can be rewritten as follows:

$$\begin{pmatrix} S_{EE} & S_{ER} & 0 \\ S_{RE} & S_{RR} & S_{RH} \\ 0 & S_{HR} & S_{HH} \end{pmatrix} \begin{pmatrix} \vec{\varphi}_E \\ \vec{\varphi}_R \\ \vec{\varphi}_H \end{pmatrix} = \begin{pmatrix} 0 \\ 0 \\ 0 \end{pmatrix}. \tag{5.3}$$

It is assumed that there are no direct connections between the electrodes and heart nodes, therefore the corresponding blocks of the system matrix are zero.

The relationship between $\vec{\varphi}_H$ and $\vec{\varphi}_E$ can be obtained from equation (5.3):

$$\vec{\varphi}_E = (S_{EE} - S_{ER}S_{RR}^{-1}S_{RE})^{-1}S_{ER}S_{RR}^{-1}S_{RH} \cdot \vec{\varphi}_H. \tag{5.4}$$

Thus the lead-field matrix can be expressed as

$$A = (S_{EE} - S_{ER}S_{RR}^{-1}S_{RE})^{-1}S_{ER}S_{RR}^{-1}S_{RH}. \tag{5.5}$$

The computation of the lead-field matrix A requires the inversion of S_{RR}. The latter includes almost the whole of the matrix S, thus the inversion may be impossible. Therefore an alternative way to compute A was developed.

Let us consider a vector $\vec{e}_i \in \mathbb{R}^n$:

$$e_{ij} = \begin{cases} 1, & j = i \\ 0, & j \neq i. \end{cases} \tag{5.6}$$

The multiplication of this vector with matrix A results in the i-th column of A. Thus setting the values of $\vec{\varphi}_H = \vec{e}_i$ and solving the problem (5.3), one can directly obtain the i-th column of the lead-field matrix. Therefore, solving the forward problem n times for each $\vec{\varphi}_H = \vec{e}_i$, the lead-field matrix can be obtained.

5.2.2 Transfer Matrix for Transmembrane Voltages

As opposed to the epi- and endocardial potentials, it is impossible to assign the TMV values to several nodes of the cardiac mesh and solve the forward problem. Since only the gradient of TMV can produce the ECG, the TMV distribution must be a steady function. For that

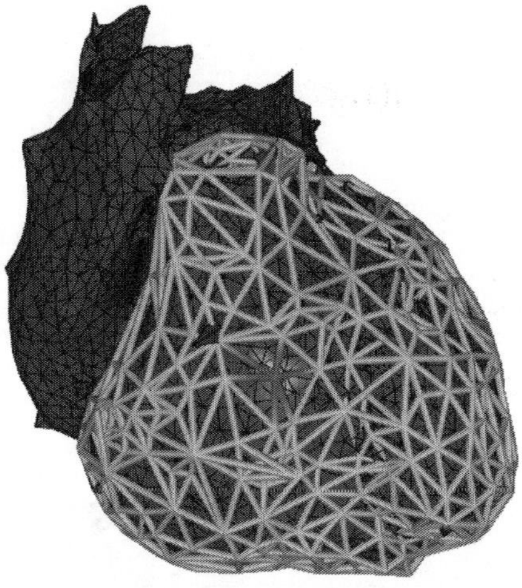

Figure 5.2: Coarse tetrahedral mesh with TMV in one node set to 1. The result of the interpolation of TMV distribution on the "fine" mesh is shown [11].

reason first a coarse mesh containing only the ventricles was introduced, with about 1000 nodes belonging to the myocardium. The TMV distributions for the computation of the transfer matrix were then defined on this coarse grid in the same manner as the node shape functions of FEM: the TMV in one node was set to 1, the rest of the nodes having the TMV of 0. These TMV distributions were interpolated to the "fine" finite element mesh where the whole forward computation could be performed (see figure 5.2).

The impressed currents were calculated from this distribution of TMV, and the forward problem was solved. The potentials on the electrodes represented a single column of the transfer matrix.

Thus the solution of the inverse problem in terms of TMV resulted in the distributions of TMV on the coarse mesh. For better visualization the interpolation of the results to the "fine" mesh was performed.

5.3 Regularization Methods

5.3.1 Singular Value Decomposition

Let us consider the singular value decomposition (SVD) of the transfer matrix A:

$$A = U\Sigma V^T = \sum_{i=1}^{r} \vec{u}_i \sigma_i \vec{v}_i^T, \qquad (5.7)$$

where $U = \{\vec{u}_1, \vec{u}_2, ..., \vec{u}_m\} \in \mathbb{R}^{m \times m}$ and $V = \{\vec{v}_1, \vec{v}_2, ..., \vec{v}_n\} \in \mathbb{R}^{n \times n}$ are matrices containing left and right eigenvectors of A correspondingly, $\Sigma = diag(\sigma_1, ..., \sigma_r)$ is a diagonal matrix containing the eigenvalues of A and $r = min(m, n)$. The properties of SVD are described in [100].

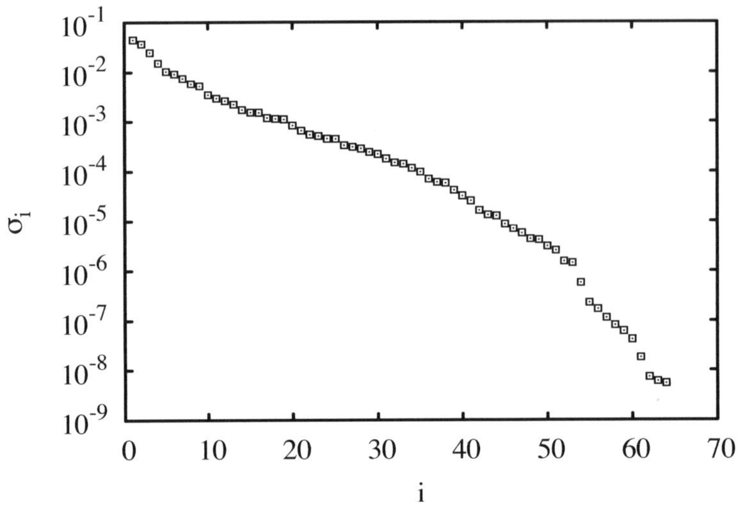

Figure 5.3: *A sample dependence of singular values of a transfer matrix σ_i on index i.*

The pseudoinverse $A^\dagger$ of the matrix A can be calculated as follows:

$$A^\dagger = \sum_{i=1}^{rank(A)} \vec{u}_i^T \frac{1}{\sigma_i} \vec{v}_i. \tag{5.8}$$

This definition of pseudoinverse can be used to compute the least squares solution of (5.2):

$$\vec{x}_{LS} = A^\dagger \vec{y} = \sum_{i=1}^{rank(A)} \frac{\vec{u}_i^T \vec{y}}{\sigma_i} \vec{v}_i, \tag{5.9}$$

which satisfies

$$\vec{x}_{LS} = \arg\min_{\vec{x}} ||A\vec{x} - \vec{y}||_2. \tag{5.10}$$

In terms of the inverse problem of electrocardiography, the vectors $\vec{u}_i$ represent a basis of the signal space, whereas the vectors $\vec{v}_i$ form a corresponding basis of the sources space [124].

The eigenvalues σ_i are usually aligned in decreasing order (see figure 5.3). The number of zero-crossings of eigenvectors $\vec{u}_i$ and $\vec{v}_i$ is growing with increasing i [100, 125], thus representing higher spatial frequencies of the measured signals as well as of the reconstructed sources. Correspondingly, the solution of (5.2) according to (5.9) results in the amplifica-

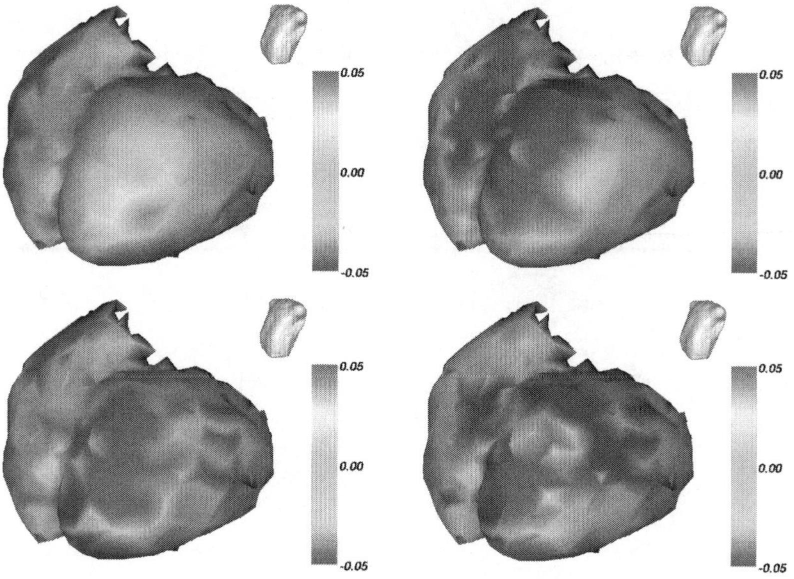

Figure 5.4: *1st (top left), 2nd (top right), 5th (bottom left) and 10th (bottom right) sources space eigenvectors of a transfer matrix. The eigenvectors with larger indices represent higher spatial frequencies.*

tion of high-frequency components of the signal. If the BSPM measurement is corrupted with noise, the solution gets unstable.

Generalized Singular Value Decomposition

The generalized singular value decomposition (GSVD) is defined for a pair of matrices $A \in \mathbb{R}^{m \times n}$ and $L \in \mathbb{R}^{p \times n}$. In terms of the inverse problem of electrocardiography, A represents the transfer matrix, and L is a regularization operator (see eq. (5.15)). Assuming that $m \geq n \geq p$, $rank(L) = p$ and the null-space of $(A^T L^T)^T$ is empty [126], the GSVD of matrices A and L can be written as follows:

$$A = U \begin{pmatrix} \Sigma & 0 \\ 0 & I_{n-p} \end{pmatrix} W^{-1}, \qquad L = V \begin{pmatrix} M & 0 \end{pmatrix} W^{-1}. \tag{5.11}$$

Matrices $U \in \mathbb{R}^{m \times n}$ and $V \in \mathbb{R}^{p \times p}$ consist of orthonormal vectors, and $W \in \mathbb{R}^{n \times n}$ is invertible with $A^T A$-orthogonal columns, i.e.

$$W^T A^T A W = \begin{pmatrix} \Sigma^2 & 0 \\ 0 & I_{n-p} \end{pmatrix}. \tag{5.12}$$

Matrices Σ and M of the size of $p \times p$ are diagonal. Their diagonal elements $\sigma_1 ... \sigma_p$ and $\mu_1 ... \mu_p$ are ordered so that

$$0 \leq \sigma_1 \leq ... \leq \sigma_p \leq 1, \qquad 1 \geq \mu_1 \geq ... \geq \mu_p \geq 0 \tag{5.13}$$

and normalized so that $\sigma_i^2 + \mu_i^2 = 1$, $i = 1..p$. Their ratios

$$\gamma_i = \frac{\sigma_i}{\mu_i}, \qquad i = 1..p \tag{5.14}$$

are referred to as generalized singular values of (A, L). According to (5.13) they are sorted in nondecreasing order.

In terms of the inverse problem of electrocardiography, the columns of matrix U make up a basis of the signal space, those of W provide the basis of the source space. As opposed to the SVD case, the basis vectors of the source space are not orthogonal.

5.3.2 Tikhonov Regularization

As it has been shown in the previous subsection, the least squares solution is unstable against high-frequency noise. Tikhonov regularization consists in the introduction of a regularization term into the formulation (5.10) [127]:

$$\vec{x}_\lambda = \arg\min_{\vec{x}}(||A\vec{x} - \vec{y}||_2^2 + \lambda^2||L\vec{x}||_2^2). \tag{5.15}$$

The regularization term $L\vec{x}$ incorporates the *a priori* information about the solution $\vec{x}$. It is assumed that the measurement noise is uncorrelated and has a diagonal covariance matrix $C_e = \epsilon^2 I$ [102], where ϵ is the scalar term and I is the unit matrix.

There are two important alternative formulations of the problem (5.15):

$$(A^T A + \lambda^2 L^T L)\vec{x} = A^T\vec{y} \tag{5.16}$$

and

$$\vec{x}_\lambda = \arg\min_{\vec{x}} \left\| \begin{pmatrix} A \\ \lambda L \end{pmatrix} \vec{x} - \begin{pmatrix} \vec{y} \\ 0 \end{pmatrix} \right\|_2. \tag{5.17}$$

Thus, if the null spaces of A and L intersect trivially such that the coefficient matrix has full rank – which is assumed implicitely throughout this chapter – then the Tikhonov solution is unique, and it can be given by

$$\vec{x}_\lambda = (A^T A + \lambda^2 L^T L)^{-1} A^T\vec{y}. \tag{5.18}$$

If matrix L is the unit matrix, the method is referred to as Tikhonov 0-order. In this case the regularization means the selection of the inverse solution with minimal 2-norm, which fulfills (5.2).

Another popular choice of matrix L is the Laplacian operator. This regularization approach is called Tikhonov 2nd order.

In terms of GSVD, the Tikhonov regularization is equivalent to the introduction of filtering factors into (5.9), suppressing the high-frequency components of the solution:

$$f_i(\lambda) = \frac{\sigma_i^2}{\sigma_i^2 + \lambda^2}, \quad L = I \quad \text{and} \quad f_i(\lambda) = \frac{\gamma_i^2}{\gamma_i^2 + \lambda^2}, \quad L \neq I. \tag{5.19}$$

Thus the solution of (5.2) can be expressed as follows:

$$\vec{x}_{reg} = \sum_{i=1}^{p} \frac{\gamma_i^2}{\gamma_i^2 + \lambda^2} \frac{\vec{u}_i^T \vec{y}}{\sigma_i} \vec{w}_i + \sum_{i=p+1}^{n} \vec{u}_i^T \vec{y} \vec{w}_i, \tag{5.20}$$

with $\vec{w}_i$ being the column vector of matrix W. If $L = I$, equation (5.20) can be reduced:

$$\vec{x}_{reg} = \sum_{i=1}^{p} \frac{\sigma_i^2}{\sigma_i^2 + \lambda^2} \frac{\vec{u}_i^T \vec{y}}{\sigma_i} \vec{v}_i. \tag{5.21}$$

5.3.3 Choice of Regularization Parameter

According to (5.20), the regularization parameter λ determines, up to which index the eigenvectors $\vec{w}_i$ can be included into the solution, that is, up to which spatial frequency the components can be considered as useful signals. If λ is chosen to be too small, the high-frequency components of (5.9) might be selected, carrying no useful information about the cardiac sources. This is called *underregularization*. On the other hand, if λ is too large, also the useful high-frequency components of the signals can be suppressed. The solution is then too smooth, and the term *overregularization* is used in this case.

Thus correct selection of the regularization parameter is extremely important for the solution of the inverse problem. Two methods were implemented to find the optimal value of λ, L-curve and CRESO.

L-curve

The L-curve is widely used to determine the optimal value of regularization parameter after the works of Hansen [102, 128]. In terms of the Tikhonov regularization, the L-curve is a parametric plot with points defined by the norm of the residual $||A\vec{x}_\lambda - \vec{y}||_2$ and the norm of the regularization term $||L\vec{x}_\lambda||_2$ for different values of the regularization parameter λ:

$$||L\vec{x}_\lambda||_2 = f(||A\vec{x}_\lambda - \vec{y}||_2). \tag{5.22}$$

This plot is usually built for λ changing within the range between the minimal and maximal eigenvalues of A. A typical L-curve for the case of measured signals $\vec{y}$ corrupted with noise is shown in figure 5.5 (solid line). The dashed line represents the L-curve for filtered $\vec{y}$, the dotted line corresponds to $\vec{y}$ containing only uncorrelated gaussian noise.

The optimal value of λ is found at the point of the maximal curvature of the L-curve, where its second derivative has its maximum. Moving the chosen λ along the curve towards the significant increase of the residual results in overregularization, whereas the movement of λ towards the increasing $||x||_2$ leads to underregularization of the solution [129].

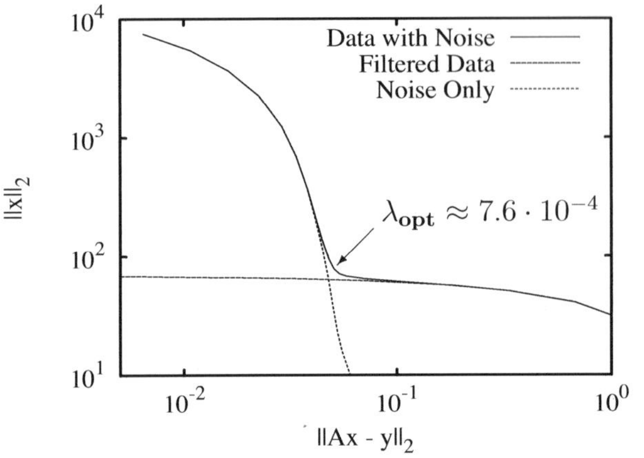

Figure 5.5: *Sample L-curves resulting from the solution of a typical inverse problem of electrocardiography. The L-curve obtained from the solution with unfiltered ECG is represented by the solid line. Dashed line corresponds to the filtered ECG, dotted line – to the pure noise. The location corresponding to the optimal λ is shown with an arrow.*

For Tikhonov 0-order regularization ($L = I$) there exist analytical formulae for the curvature of the L-curve [11, 128].

According to [128], the L-curve criterion delivers a good estimation for the optimal value of the regularization parameter even in the case of correlated noise in $\vec{y}$, thus being the method of choice if the transfer matrix A is corrupted by modeling errors.

CRESO

The method of composite residual and smoothing operator (CRESO) consists in the localization of the maximum of the following function:

$$C(\lambda) = ||\vec{x}_\lambda||_2^2 + 2\lambda^2 \frac{d}{d(\lambda^2)} ||\vec{x}_\lambda||_2^2. \tag{5.23}$$

The case of Tikhonov 0-order regularization is assumed.

If the SVD of A is known, $C(\lambda)$ can be computed as

$$C(\lambda) = \sum_{i=1}^{rank(A)} \left(\frac{\sigma_i}{\sigma_i^2 + \lambda^2} \vec{u}_i^T \vec{y} \right)^2 \cdot \left(1 - \frac{4\lambda^2}{\sigma_i^2 + \lambda^2} \right). \tag{5.24}$$

Figure 5.6 shows a sample CRESO curve; the data used for the inverse problem solution correspond to those shown in figure 5.5, for the case of BSPM corrupted with noise.

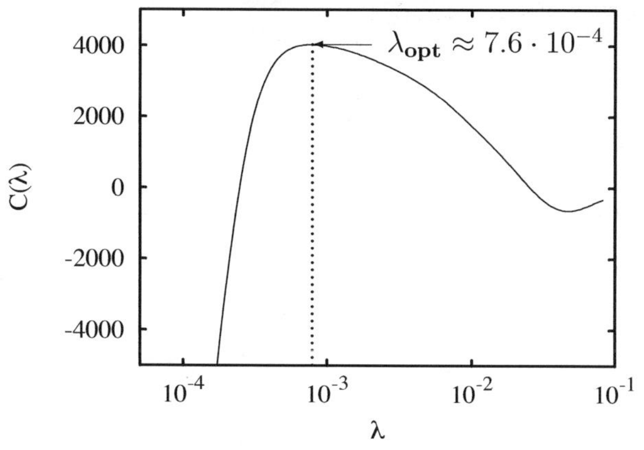

Figure 5.6: *A sample CRESO curve for the same problem as shown in figure 5.5. The case of BSPM corrupted with noise is shown.*

The computation times necessary to find the optimal value of the regularization parameter is comparable for both methods. The values of optimal λ delivered by both methods are quite near.

5.3.4 Maximum A Posteriori Estimation

The regularization method of maximum a posteriori estimation (MAP) employs a statistical basis of *a priori* estimations of the inverse problem solutions and chooses the best solution fitting the given observation $\vec{y}$ out of it. This approach is based on the theory developed by Foster in [130].

Let's assume the considered (forward) problem is expressed as follows (cf. equation (5.2)):

$$\vec{y} = A\vec{x} + \vec{e}, \tag{5.25}$$

where $\vec{e}$ is the vector of random measurement errors, presumed to have zero mean and known covariances [131]. The goal is to construct a matrix operator $H \in \mathbb{R}^{n \times m}$ such that the averages

$$\vec{x}\,' = H\vec{y} \tag{5.26}$$

would represent the best possible solution of (5.25). Combining (5.25) and (5.26) we obtain

$$\vec{x}\,' = HA\vec{x} + H\vec{e} = R\vec{x} + H\vec{e}, \tag{5.27}$$

where the rows of the matrix $R = HA$ represent a set of filters transforming the exact solution $\vec{x}$ to our estimation $\vec{x}'$ minus some random error.

If the exact solution $\vec{x}$ is subtracted from the both sides of equation (5.27), the estimation error can be obtained:

$$\vec{x}' - \vec{x} = (HA - I)\vec{x} + H\vec{e}. \tag{5.28}$$

The first term at the right side of (5.28) is usually referred to as a resolving error or *bias*, whereas the second term represents random error. If $\vec{x}'$ provides a reasonable estimation of $\vec{x}$, both of these terms must be small.

Given a statistical description for the variability of $\vec{x}$ in the form of covariance matrix C_x, and assuming that the errors in the *a priori* estimate $\vec{x}_0$ are statistically independent on the data errors $\vec{e}$, the covariance of estimation errors $\vec{x}' - \vec{x}$ can be represented as

$$C = (HA - I)C_x(HA - I)^T + HC_eH^T. \tag{5.29}$$

The first term is the covariance of resolving errors, the second term represents the covariance of random errors "projected" into the estimates of the data. The estimator which minimizes the diagonal elements of C in (5.29) is

$$H = C_xA^T(AC_xA^T + C_e)^{-1}, \tag{5.30}$$

which is also known as the "minimal variance" estimator. This equation was originally derived in [132] as the best linear estimator when $\vec{x}$ is a realization of a second-order gaussian random process. Still the assumption of gaussian distribution is not necessary, the variance of estimation errors can be minimized by (5.30) regardless of the form of *a priori* probability density of $\vec{x}$.

In this way an estimate of $\vec{x}$ can be obtained:

$$\vec{x}' = C_xA^T(AC_xA^T + C_e)^{-1}\vec{y}, \tag{5.31}$$

which is used as the solution of the inverse problem.

This method was employed by van Oosterom in [133] to reconstruct the potential distributions on the cardiac surface. The *a priori* data were generated using the UDL approach (see section 5.1) from reconstructed activation times during the QRS-complex. These data represented a matrix Ψ_r with the potentials on the nodes of a "pericardial" mesh saved in columns and the change of the potential in a single node in rows. The spatial covariance matrix of *a priori* estimation was defined as

$$C_x = \frac{1}{N}\Psi_r\Psi_r^T, \tag{5.32}$$

where N represented the number of time samples in the matrix Ψ_r. The covariance matrix of random errors C_e was approximated with λI.

The results obtained using this method were compared with those obtained from Tikhonov 0-order, Tikhonov 2-order and truncated SVD approaches. The relative error for the MAP-based method was shown to be up to 5 times smaller than the rest for different levels of induced noise.

This method has been implemented in the course of current research and tested with several patient data sets [134, 135].

Based on the MAP regularization, a Bayesian methodology to solve the inverse problem of electrocardiography was recently developed [136, 137].

5.3.5 Spatiotemporal MAP-Regularization

Spatial MAP-regularization considers vectors $\vec{x}$ and $\vec{y}$ in equation (5.25) as the distributions of cardiac sources and BSPM in a given time instant, respectively. The time instants are considered independently, although the value of, say, transmembrane voltage in a given point generally depends on the value of TMV in this point at previous time instants. This important information is not used for stabilization of the inverse problem.

Thus an alternative approach has been developed in the course of the current work [138, 139, 140]. Vectors $\vec{x}$, $\vec{y}$ and $\vec{e}$ in (5.25) are replaced with compound column vectors $\tilde{\vec{x}}$, $\tilde{\vec{y}}$ and $\tilde{\vec{e}}$ containing the corresponding distributions at multiple (typically neighboring) time instants. The transfer matrix A is replaced with a "diagonal block matrix" $\tilde{A}$:

$$\begin{pmatrix} A & 0 & \dots & 0 \\ 0 & A & \dots & 0 \\ \vdots & \vdots & \ddots & \vdots \\ 0 & 0 & \dots & A \end{pmatrix} \begin{pmatrix} \vec{x}_1 \\ \vec{x}_2 \\ \vdots \\ \vec{x}_N \end{pmatrix} = \begin{pmatrix} \vec{y}_1 \\ \vec{y}_2 \\ \vdots \\ \vec{y}_N \end{pmatrix} + \begin{pmatrix} \vec{e}_1 \\ \vec{e}_2 \\ \vdots \\ \vec{e}_N \end{pmatrix}, \tag{5.33}$$

or

$$\tilde{\vec{y}} = \tilde{A}\tilde{\vec{x}} + \tilde{\vec{e}}. \tag{5.34}$$

Here N is the number of simultaneously considered time instants. The further solution does not differ from the method described in the previous subsection. The amount of RAM consumed by this method is therefore larger than that for the purely spatial MAP-regularization, but the quality of delivered results is strongly improved due to a larger amount of *a priori* information employed.

5.3.6 Assumption of Monotonically Changing Transmembrane Voltage

This temporal constraint on the solution of the inverse problem has been proposed by the group of Tilg in [117]. This approach is based on the fact that the basic form of an action potential is well known. During the depolarization of the cardiac tissue it can be assumed that the value of TMV in each point never decreases. Although this assumption is not quite correct (see, e.g., action potential curves in figure 7.3), the start-up pike of an action potential curve caused by the fast Na^+ current due to its small size does not affect the resulting ECG strongly.

The assumption of nondecreasing TMV can be mathematically expressed as follows:

$$\vec{x}_{min} \leq \vec{x}_1 \leq \vec{x}_2 \leq \ldots \leq \vec{x}_{max}, \tag{5.35}$$

where $\vec{x}_{min}$ and $\vec{x}_{max}$ represent the smallest and largest possible TMV values, respectively. These constraints can be written in matrix form:

$$\begin{pmatrix} -\vec{x}_1 \\ \vec{x}_1 - \vec{x}_2 \\ \vdots \\ \vec{x}_{N-1} - \vec{x}_N \\ \vec{x}_N \end{pmatrix} \leq \begin{pmatrix} -\vec{x}_{min} \\ 0 \\ \vdots \\ 0 \\ \vec{x}_{max} \end{pmatrix}. \tag{5.36}$$

This is an important constraint which strongly improves the quality of solution of equation (5.33) for the QRS-complex.

Similar operations can be performed for the assumption of nonincreasing TMV during the repolarization phase of the heart cycle.

5.3.7 Generalized Minimal Residual (GMRes)

The application of GMRes approach to the solution of ill-posed inverse problems was considered by Calvetti in [141]. Afterwards this method was applied to the inverse problem of electrocardiography in [142].

The GMRes method belongs to the class of iterative regularization methods. It is assumed in this method, that the transfer matrix is square. Therefore for the purpose of the present work equation (5.2) can be transformed as follows:

$$A^T \cdot A \cdot \vec{x} = A^T \cdot \vec{y}. \tag{5.37}$$

Matrix $A' = A^T \cdot A$ is square and symmetric. The right-hand vector of measured body surface potentials $\vec{y}$ is replaced with $\vec{b} = A^T \cdot \vec{y}$. Substituting these changes into (5.37), we obtain

$$A' \cdot \vec{x} = \vec{b}. \tag{5.38}$$

The solution is found in an orthonormal basis, which is formed using an Arnoldi process [143] in the Krylov space [144]. In each iteration a new basis vector is built. The projections of the solution on these basis vectors are sought, which minimize the residual $||A'\vec{x} - \vec{b}||_2$. The exact iterative algorithm can be found in [100, 141, 145].

An important feature of GMRes consists in the divergence of the solution from the desired values after some iteration step (see figure 5.7). Therefore a criterion is required to determine the optimal number of iterations in each case. In [141] a variation of the L-curve method is proposed, with the number of iterations considered as regularization parameter.

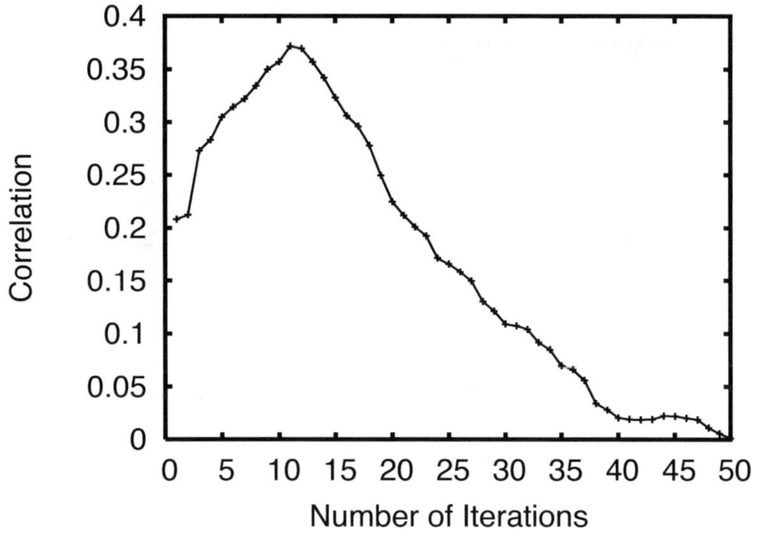

Figure 5.7: *The dependence of correlation between simulated and reconstructed heart surface potentials on the number of GMRes iterations. The solution starts diverging from the original data after the 12th iteration.*

5.3.8 Greensite Spatiotemporal Approach

The usage of the spatial regularization algorithms presumes that in each time instant the sources are reconstructed separately. Thus the spatio-temporal nature of the ECG signal is neglected. Therefore a new approach was developed by Greensite in [146], allowing to modify the regularization methods described above in order to take this nature into account.

This approach consists in the computation of SVD of the matrix Y with rows containing the change of potential in a single lead of ECG, and columns containing the BSPM in each time instant:

$$Y = PQT^T, \tag{5.39}$$

where the matrix P contains the spatial eigenvectors of Y, T the temporal ones and Q is a diagonal matrix containing the eigenvalues of Y (cf. equation (5.7)). The notation used here is taken from [118]. Let's re-write the equation (5.2) as follows:

$$A \cdot X = Y, \tag{5.40}$$

where X is a matrix the columns of which represent the distributions of cardiac sources $\vec{x}$ in all the time instants. Substituting (5.39) into (5.40) and multiplying both sides by T results in

$$A \cdot X \cdot T = P \cdot Q. \tag{5.41}$$

The matrix product $X \cdot T$ can be replaced with Ξ denoting the matrix of new unknowns:

$$A \cdot \Xi = P \cdot Q. \tag{5.42}$$

In the system (5.42) only first several equations satisfying the discrete Picard conditions [102] are considered. The inverse problem of electrocardiography is solved in terms of the matrix of unknowns Ξ. Multiplying it by T^T, the matrix of solutions X can be obtained afterwards. It has been shown in [146], that this approach leads to more accurate reconstruction results. The same conclusion has been made in the course of the present work.

Chapter 6

Patient Data Acquisition

6.1 Patients

Information about 8 subjects was acquired within the scope of the project [147] supported by the German Research Association (Deutsche Forschungsgemeinschaft, DFG). The aim of the project was to develop novel quantitative methods of noninvasive diagnostics of cardiac diseases with special emphasis on the repolarization phase. The data sets for each patient included an MRI scan of the patient's thorax and heart as well as a multichannel ECG. Table 6.1 contains a short summary of the involved subjects.

The first data set was made for training purposes: a healthy subject was involved. This measurement was performed in order to work out the workflow of data acquisition, develop the software necessary for the processing of measured data and test the reconstruction strategy. Also the difference between the reconstruction results computed for the healthy subject and those for a patient suffering from some cardiac disease would better reveal the pathological features.

Further on seven data sets were created for patients suffering from various heart diseases. These include posterior (pat. 001), posterolateral (002) as well as anterior (004,007) infarctions, myocarditis (003) and left bundle branch block (005). The infarction location for patient 006 is not known.

6.2 Anatomical Model

The acquisition of MRI data was performed using a Siemens Magnetom Vision scanner at the University Hospital of Würzburg, Germany. The magnetic field strength of this scanner was 1.5 T. At least two data sets were acquired for each patient, one for the whole thorax and one for the heart in the diastolic phase. For two patients also a data set for the heart in the systolic phase was created.

The FLASH 3D gradient pulse sequence was used for all the data sets [148, 149]. This sequence is characterized by flip angles far below 90°, typically of 15°. Thus a strong reduction of the repetition time – and, correspondingly, of the recording duration – was achieved.

Pat. ID	Initials	Sex	Age	Diagnosis
Prob001	M. H.	M	20	Healthy
001	E. L.	M	63	Posterior Infarction 6/89
002	P. K.	M	61	Posterolateral Infarction 8/03, Posterior Infarction 00
003	H. S.	M	43	Myocarditis, DCM, ICD-Impl.
004	P. H.	M	54	Anterior Infarction 04/03
005	W. O.	M	46	Left Bundle Branch Block
006	G. M.	F	67	Infarction
007	A. Z.	M	48	Anterior Infarction

Table 6.1: *List of subjects involved into the measurements. Their initials, sex, age and clinical diagnosis are shown.*

The data set for the torso of the patient was made up from a sequence of frontal images with the typical resolution of $4 \times 4 \times 4\ mm^3$. The recording time for this data set was 40 s, so the recordings were made in breath-hold, which reduced the artifacts of the images.

The patient's heart was recorded by a set of short axis plane (SAX) images. The repetition time was 230 ms, echo time 2.7 ms. The imaging was ECG-triggered, so the images of the heart in a preselected phase could be obtained. The overall recording time for each heart phase was about 11 min, the resolution was about $2 \times 2 \times 4\ mm^3$. An example of SAX scan is shown in figure 6.1.

In order to perform the segmentation of these data sets, the methods described in section 3.1 were employed.

6.3 ECG Acquisition and Processing

6.3.1 ECG Acquisition

The ECGs of the patients were acquired using an *ActiveTwo* ECG measuring device with 64 leads manufactured by BioSemi, the Netherlands. This system contains an ADC with 24-bit dynamic range. The electrodes are attached to the thorax of a patient as shown in figure 6.2. Their coordinates are registered using a Polhemus Fastrak localization system (Polhemus Inc., Vermont, USA).

Each electrode of the BioSemi system possesses its own signal amplifier - *active electrodes*. This approach has increased the signal-to-noise ratio (SNR) of the measurements. The main amplifier is battery-based, which reduced the interferences of the signal with the power line frequency.

The sample rate for the ECG measurements is typically set to 2048 Hz. The 50 Hz power line noise is suppressed using a built-in hardware filter of the ActiveTwo system. The recording time was 200 s.

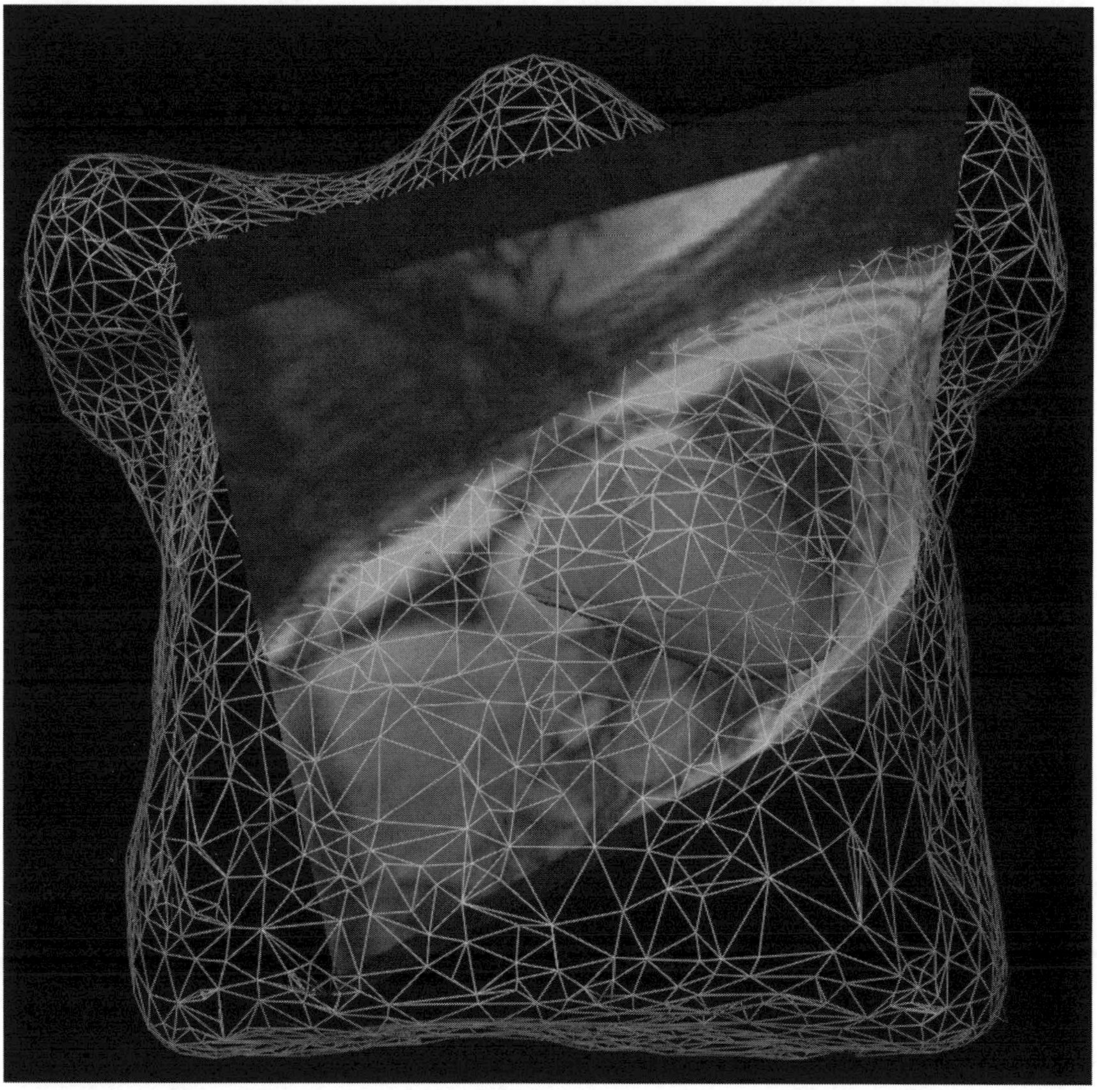

Figure 6.1: *An example SAX-image of the heart. The contours of the heart segmented from the same data set as well as the torso are shown for better orientation.*

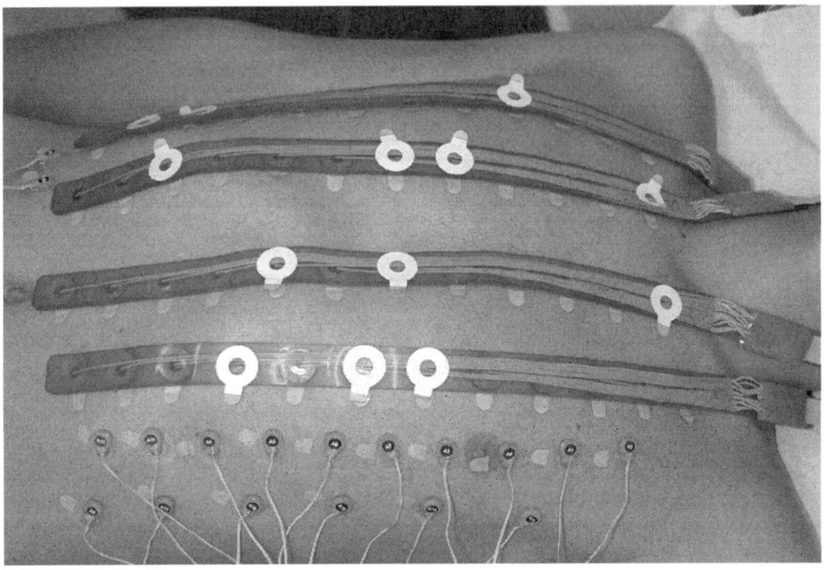

Figure 6.2: *64 electrodes attached to the thorax of a patient*

The data from the BioSemi system are acquired by a special program supplied with the system. This program is able to visualize the measured ECG in real time and to save the recorded data in its own format onto the hard disc of a PC.

6.3.2 ECG Filtering

A special software tool was written, capable to read the data from the files saved by BioSemi software and to apply different filtering methods. This tool employs the AltiVec unit of PowerPC G4/G5 processors in order to speed up the calculations. The filtering methods implemented in this software are listed below.

Fourier Filtering

This filtering method was used, if the beat-to-beat variation of the ECG signal and of the RR-interval was relatively large. Another important application of this approach was to investigate the extrasystolic beats.

A fast Fourier transform is applied to the whole recording sequence of each channel (typically around 4×10^5 samples). Afterwards a bandpass filter is applied, suppressing the components of the signal with too low and too high frequencies. The lower cut-off frequency is normally set to 0.06 Hz, the higher one to 200 Hz. The user can choose between the box, Bartlett and Hann border of the bandpass [150]. Also the harmonics of 50 Hz caused by the interference with the power line frequency are suppressed.

The result of such filtering needs additional baseline correction. The user is able to define the time offsets relative to the R-peak, at which the ECG signal is assumed to be zero. The values of 10 samples around the given point are averaged in order to obtain a more precise baseline offset. The baseline between these points is linearly interpolated and subtracted from the ECG signal.

The disadvantage of Fourier filtering consists in the impossibility to separate the signal from noise only by their frequencies. Therefore another method to get rid of uncorrelated noise was proposed.

Averaging Multiple ECG Cycles

If the heart rate is constant during the whole measurement, it is possible in each channel to cut out all the ECG cycles, superimpose them and compute the average. Thus the uncorrelated noise is suppressed (the signal-to-noise ratio is increased by the factor of $\sqrt{N}$, where N is the number of superimposed cycles).

Three different approaches to choose the interval being averaged as well as the averaging method are proposed by the program.

1. Averaged is the interval between the neighboring R-peaks. As all the RR-intervals have different length, the linear interpolation is chosen to find out the corresponding points. This method was abandoned because of the high computation cost, complicated baseline correction and a large variation of the T-wave position.

2. Hausdorff averaging is used as described in [151]. The phase space of the ECG is built, in which each cycle is represented by a closed loop. One can exactly distinguish the phases of the ECG and perform averaging for the given interval of phases. This method appeared to be very sensitive against noise, therefore introducing a large distortion into the signal.

3. The user can define the limits of the averaged interval relatively to the R-peak position (say, -200 till +600 ms). At the borders of this interval the ECG signal is assumed to be zero. All superimposed intervals have the same length, so the averaging and baseline correction can be easily performed. This method is the choice for virtually all measurements.

R-Peak Detection

An important part of the filtering methods described above is R-peak detection. A simple but rather reliable method has been developed, which is able to find almost 100% of the R-peaks in all the provided ECG records.

The following steps are done to perform the R-peak detection. First, the Fourier-filter is applied on the ECG signal in the chosen channel with the bandpass frequency range of 0.06-75 Hz and the suppression of 50 Hz. Then the second derivative of the filtered signal is computed. Its maximal value is found, and a threshold value is computed by multiplication of the maximal value with a user-defined factor (typically 0.3). Afterwards the array is checked to find the first data point having the second derivative higher than the threshold.

This point is considered as the onset of the R-peak. The offset of the R-peak is similarly sought starting from the time point of the onset+200 ms and then moving backward. The R-peak is assumed to be located exactly between these two points.

The user is able to change the threshold, thus assuring the correct detection of all the R-peaks in the given channel and simultaneously avoiding the erroneous detection of the other peaks.

The R-peaks found in the selected channel are used for filtering of all the other channels, which significantly improves the overall performance. Also the reliability of the detection is improved, because the channel with the best SNR can be selected to determine the R-peak locations.

Advanced ECG Filtering and R-Peak Detection Methods

A large number of advanced filtering and R-peak detection methods were developed at the Institute of Biomedical Engineering, Universität Karlsruhe (TH) during the course of this work by the group of Antoun Khawaja [152, 153, 154, 155]. They are to be integrated to the signal analysis of this work in future.

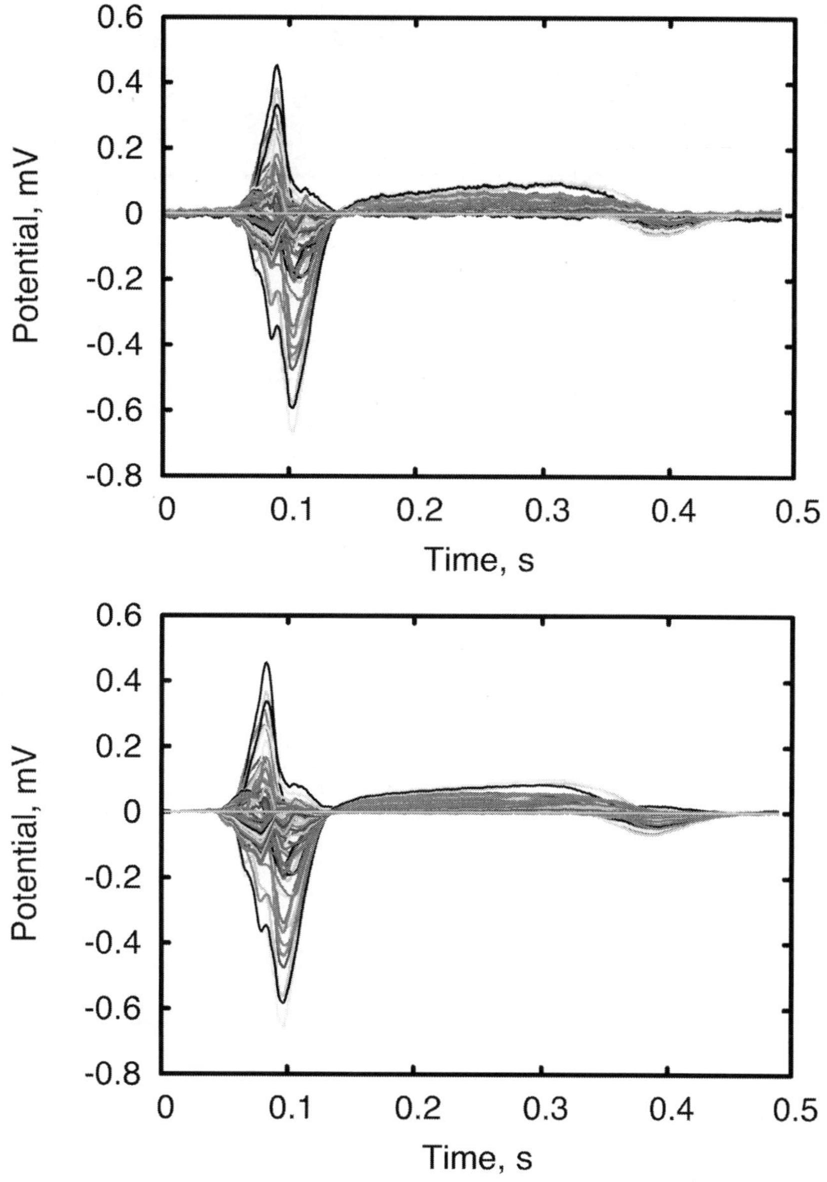

Figure 6.3: *64 ECG leads measured on a patient: before filtering (the average value was subtracted in each channel, top), after averaging over 200 ECG cycles (bottom). A QRST-complex is shown.*

Chapter 7

Modeling of the Patient's Heart

7.1 Anatomical Model of the Heart Including Excitation Conduction System

The anatomical model of the patient's heart was created based on the provided short axis MRI scan representing the diastolic phase of the heart. Deformable triangle meshes were used to segment both ventricles from this scan, as described in section 6.2.

As the SAX-images of the heart did not contain atria, and the resolution of the thorax images was not high enough to segment them, they were replaced by a region containing blood with the shape roughly corresponding to that of the atria. Thus the conductivity distribution within the thorax was kept, although the P-wave of the ECG could not be simulated properly. Correspondingly, the SA-node was not included into the model, so the main pacemaking unit was the AV-node. The anatomy of the heart was defined on a regular grid with the resolution of $1 \times 1 \times 1\ mm^3$.

The excitation conduction system was implemented as a tree-like structure originating from the AV-node. It was subdivided into two branches. One of them was going along the septum towards the apex of the right ventricle (right Tawara bundle). Another branch was put into the left ventricle and there split once again into the left anterior and left posterior fascicles. The conduction of excitation between these branches and the ventricular myocardium was disabled.

An automatic process generated a set of nodes on the inner surface of the ventricles and connected them into the trees representing the Purkinje fibers. These fibers were attached to the free endings of the former three branches. The function of the Purkinje fibers was to carry the excitation from the apex towards the base of the ventricles, distributing it throughout the endocardium. A typical heart model including the left and right ventricles, blood and excitation conduction system is shown in figure 7.1.

The anatomical model of the heart is described in [156] in more detail.

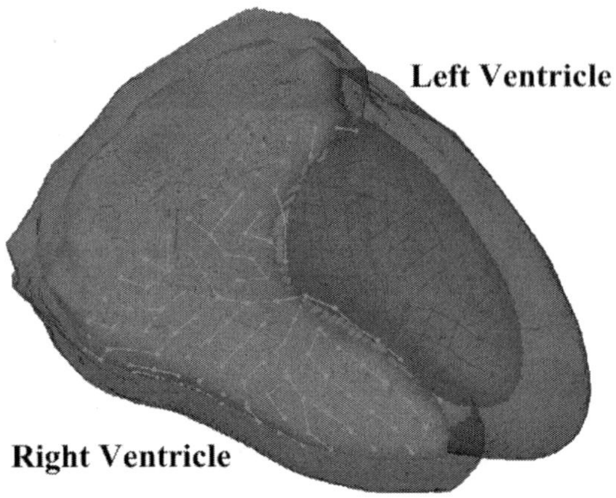

Figure 7.1: *The anatomical model of the patient's heart. Left and right ventricles, blood inside them as well as excitation conduction system are shown.*

Tissue Class	Longitudinal ECV, mm/s	Anisotropy Ratio
Left ventricular myocardium	1200	3
Right ventricular myocardium	1200	3
Right Tawara branch	2250	1
Left anterior fascicle	2000	1
Left posterior fascicle	2000	1
Right Purkinje fibers	4860	1
Left Purkinje fibers	3310	1

Table 7.1: *The default values of excitation conduction velocity (ECV) for different tissue classes within the heart. Anisotropy ratio represents the ratio between longitudinal (along the fiber orientation) and transversal (perpendicular to the fiber orientation) ECVs. As the excitation conduction system is represented by a tree-like structure, there is no need to introduce the anisotropy of ECV for it.*

7.2 Modeling of the Depolarization Phase

The QRS-complex of ECG is formed by the propagation of the depolarization front through the ventricular myocardium. This propagation is defined by the geometry of the heart as well as by the distribution of excitation conduction velocities within the heart. As the anatomical cardiac model contains several different tissue types, parameters of which can be varied, it is possible to fine-tune the depolarization sequence of the ventricles. Tissue classes for which the excitation conduction velocities (ECVs) are varied as well as the default values of ECVs are shown in Table 7.1.

In the case of anisotropic ECVs the corresponding anisotropy ratios were kept constant during the optimization, with each component of ECV being multiplied by the same factor.

The default values of ECV for the excitation conduction system were adapted from [52], for the ventricular myocardium it was computed using the ten Tusscher cell model [22].

The diseases influencing the depolarization sequence as well as the way these diseases have been modelled are described in detail in Section 7.4.

7.3 Dispersion of Action Potential Duration

7.3.1 Transmural APD Dispersion

The ten Tusscher cell model has already incorporated the transmural dispersion of myocyte properties [22]. This model was employed to generate the action potential curves to be used with the cellular automaton.

The number of different types of myocardial tissue is set to 97, with the first one describing endocardium, and the last one corresponding to epicardium. For each tissue type, its own conductivities for various transmembrane ionic currents are defined according to [22]. A transmural patch of ventricular myocardium is created including all 97 tissue types (see figure 7.2), in order to introduce the intercellular coupling into the model. The voxel size in this patch was $0.2 \times 0.2 \times 0.2\ mm^3$, the overall size of the patch was $9 \times 9 \times 117$ voxels, or $1.8 \times 1.8 \times 23.4\ mm^3$, with tissue index changing along the z axis. At the endocardial side of the patch, a periodical excitation is applied simulating the signals coming from the Purkinje fibers in the real heart. The frequency of excitation is varied in order to investigate the response of APD on this variation. The TMV in each layer of the patch is recorded for the whole excitation cycle, thus forming an action potential curve for each tissue type. Such a family of curves corresponding to the excitation frequency of 1 Hz (60 beats per minute) is shown in figure 7.3.

Three parameters are used to vary the transmural dispersion of APD, representing scaling coefficients for endocardial, midmyocardial and epicardial APD (p_{endo}, p_m and p_{epi}). These parameters are allowed to change only within the range between 0.7 and 1.3. The modified APD for the i-th action potential curve ($i \in 0..96$) is calculated using the following equation:

$$APD_i = \begin{cases} APD_i^0 \cdot (p_{endo} + (p_m - p_{endo}) \sin(3\pi i/192)) & \text{for } i < 32 \\ APD_i^0 \cdot (p_{epi} + (p_m - p_{epi}) \cos(3\pi (i-32)/384)) & \text{for } i >= 32 \end{cases} \qquad (7.1)$$

An example transmural distribution of scaling factors with $p_{endo} = 1$, $p_m = 1.2$ and $p_{epi} = 0.9$ is shown in figure 7.4.

7.3.2 Gradient of APD

Another form of the APD dispersion considered in this work was a single gradient of APD defined for the whole ventricular myocardium. It was defined by 4 parameters: azimuth and declination in the own coordinate system of the left ventricle, defining the orientation of the vector; the change of APD per millimeter along the vector, defining the magnitude of dispersion; and the APD in the center of coordinates.

Figure 7.2: A transmural patch of myocardial tissue, with excitation applied at endocardium. The frequency of excitation was 1 Hz. Time after the last excitation for each figure, top to bottom: 6, 12, 18, 24, 226, 289, 310 ms.

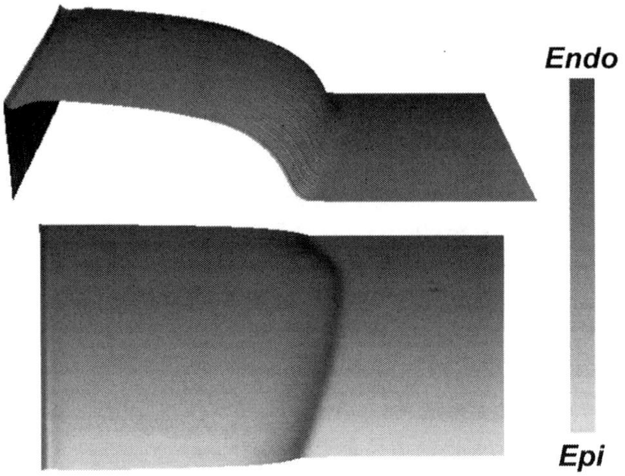

Figure 7.3: A family of 97 action potential curves representing the response of different types of ventricular myocardium (from endo- till epicardium) on the external stimulation with the frequency of 1 Hz. Each curve was recorded during 512 ms.

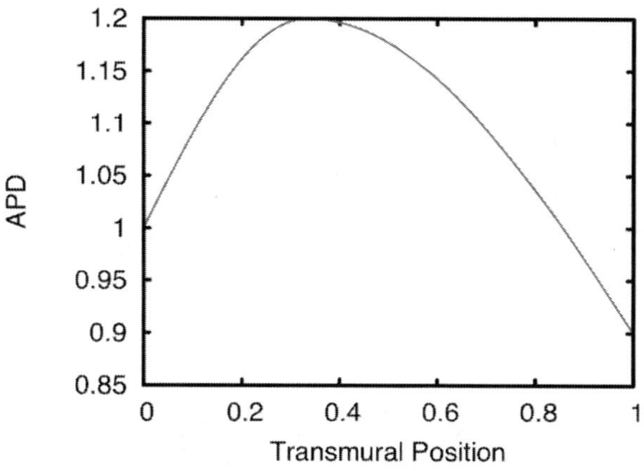

Figure 7.4: *An example distribution of scaling factors across the ventricular wall with* $p_{endo} = 1$, $p_m = 1.2$ *and* $p_{epi} = 0.9$.

The introduction of a single gradient of action potential duration cannot describe a complicated APD distribution like that obtained in [33]. Still, if used together with the transmural dispersion of APD, it can deliver quite good correspondence between the simulated and measured ECG (see section 8.3).

7.3.3 APD in Segments

As it has already been mentioned, a single gradient of APD might not be able to describe the real APD dispersion in the human heart, which could be quite complicated. Therefore another approach to define this dispersion has been developed.

First, APD is defined in several locations of the heart model. Afterwards a tetrahedron mesh is created, with nodes located in these points as well as at the corners of the bounding box defining the borders of the data set. The distribution of APD is then linearly interpolated on the whole heart using the node shape functions described in section 4.3.

A set of 10 standard locations has been defined in the own coordinate system of the left ventricle. This set was the same for all the hearts considered within the scope of the current work. Their locations are defined by their azimuths and declinations, as shown in table 7.2.

Point Number	Asimuth φ	Declination θ
1	0	$\pi/9$
2	π	$\pi/9$
3	0	$\pi/3$
4	$\pi/2$	$\pi/3$
5	π	$\pi/3$
6	$3 \cdot \pi/2$	$\pi/3$
7	0	$11 \cdot \pi/18$
8	$\pi/2$	$11 \cdot \pi/18$
9	π	$11 \cdot \pi/18$
10	$3 \cdot \pi/2$	$11 \cdot \pi/18$

Table 7.2: *Coordinates of the anchor points were the APD is defined. The angles are set in the own coordinate system of the left ventricle. If the ray in the given direction anywhere crosses the right ventricle, the point is chosen in the right ventricle.*

7.4 Modeling of Specific Heart Diseases

7.4.1 Infarction and Ischemia

An infarction scar can be introduced into the model of the patient's heart as a spherical region, where the amplitude of the action potential as well as the excitation conduction velocity of each voxel are suppressed. The APD in the voxels with ischemic tissue is decreased as well. A typical dependency of these parameters on the distance between the given voxel and the center of infarction is shown in figure 7.5.

The site and size of the infarction scar are controlled by the following 5 parameters:

- the azimuth of the center of infarction scar in the own coordinate system of the left ventricle;
- the declination of the center of infarction scar in this coordinate system;
- the distance between the center of infarction and the endocardium along this axis normalized by the radius of infarction;
- the radius of infarction area in mm;
- the thickness of the border zone of infarction scar (see figure 7.5).

The influence of the infarction on the cells at the surface of the ventricle (and thus the possibility of excitation to be conducted by the Purkinje fibers within the area of infarction) can be controlled by the user (see figure 7.6). The ECGs simulated for a patient with an infarction are shown in figure 7.9.

According to [7], the extracellular conductivity of myocardial tissue increases within the area of infarction scar. On the other hand, the intracellular conductivity within this region should be reduced due to the closure of intercellular gap junctions. Both of these

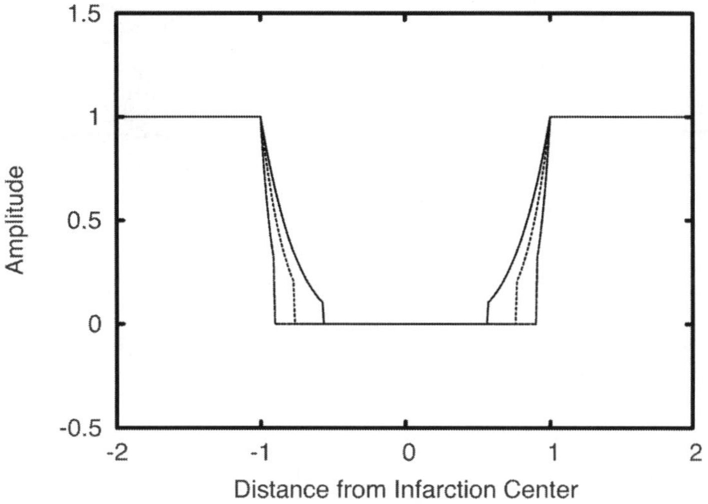

Figure 7.5: *The dependencies of action potential amplitude, excitation conduction velocity and action potential duration on the distance to the center of infarction defined for different sizes of the border zone between infarcted and healthy tissues.*

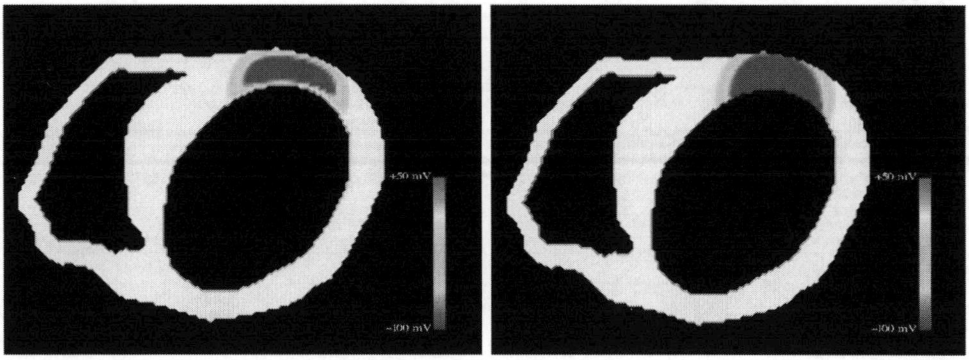

Figure 7.6: *Distributions of transmembrane voltages in the middle of ST-segment for a heart with infarction. The influence of infarction on the surface of the heart can be changed by the user. In the left case the impact factor is set to 0, in the right case to 1.*

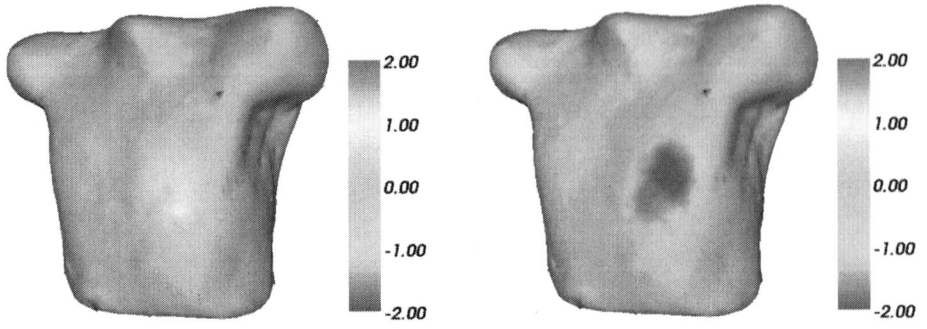

Figure 7.7: *Body surface potential maps corresponding to the TMV distributions shown in figure 7.6. The elevation of the ST-segment in the case of the impact factor 0 (left) is caused only by the unequal anisotropy ratio (see section 8.1) and disappears in the case of equal anisotropy ratio. The potentials are shown in mV.*

processes were taken into account while the simulated ECGs for infarcted patients were built.

7.4.2 Bundle Branch Block

A block of each bundle branch can be introduced by disconnecting the nodes of the tree-shaped excitation conduction system (see Section 7.1). Thus, a block of the left Tawara bundle branch, for instance, results in a significant delay of excitation of the left ventricle. The depolarization front needs to pass through the septum in order to reach the left endocardium. There it can perform a re-excitation of the Purkinje fibers, the latter carry the excitation throughout the endocardium of the left ventricle. The transmembrane voltage distributions simulated for a healthy heart, for a heart with a left bundle branch block and a heart with infarction are compared in figure 7.8, the ECGs for these three cases are compared in figure 7.9.

7.4.3 Extrasystolic Beats

The modeling of extrasystolic beats can be performed by introduction of spontaneous excitation centers into the ventricular myocardium. The excitation is conducted by the myocardium to the excitation conduction system, which rapidly propagates it throughout the ventricles. The distributions of transmembrane voltages during an extrasystolic beat with a spontaneous excitation center located on the left ventricular lateral wall is shown in figure 7.10. The corresponding multichannel ECG is indicated in figure 7.11.

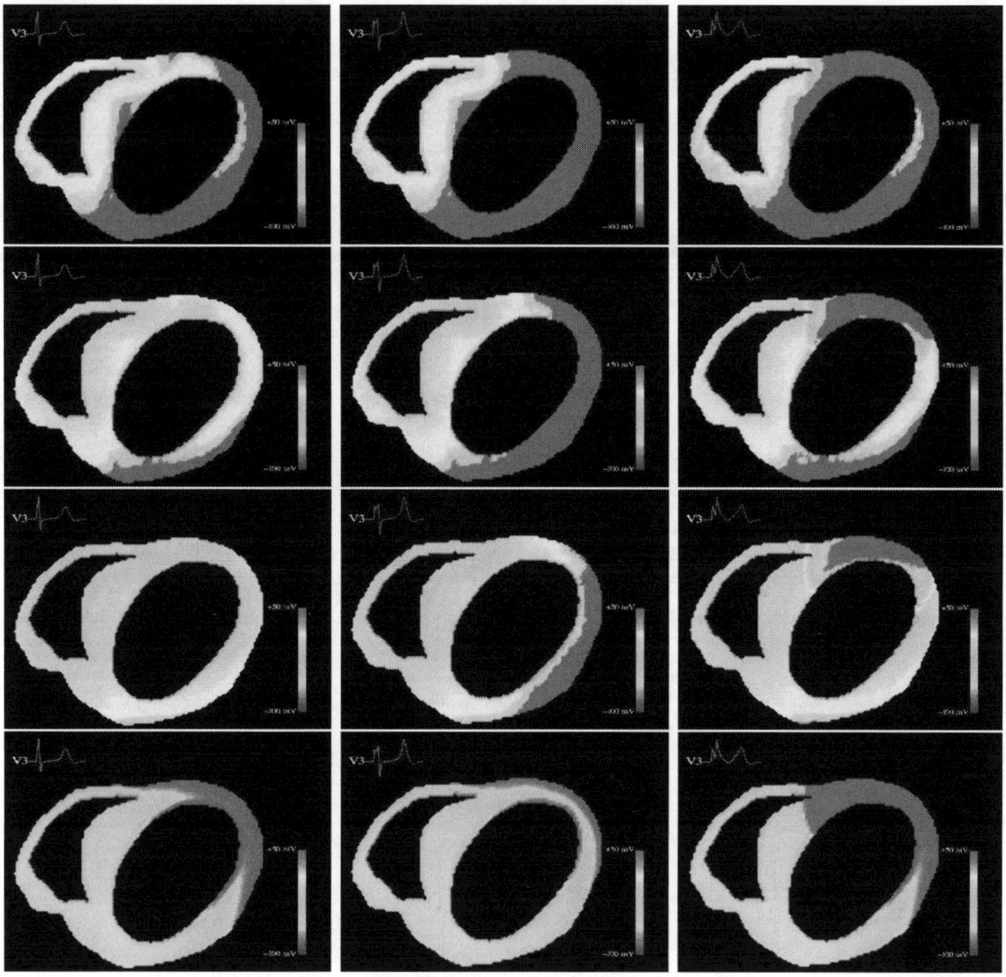

Figure 7.8: *Distributions of transmembrane voltages in a healthy heart (left), a heart with left bundle branch block (center) and a heart with anterior infarction (right). Corresponding phases of the ECG is shown in the upper left corner of each picture.*

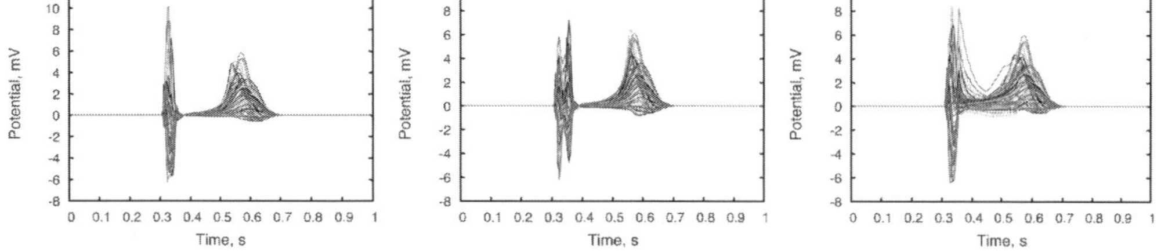

Figure 7.9: *64 channels of simulated ECG for a healthy heart (left), a heart with left bundle branch block (center) and a heart with anterior myocardial infarction (right).*

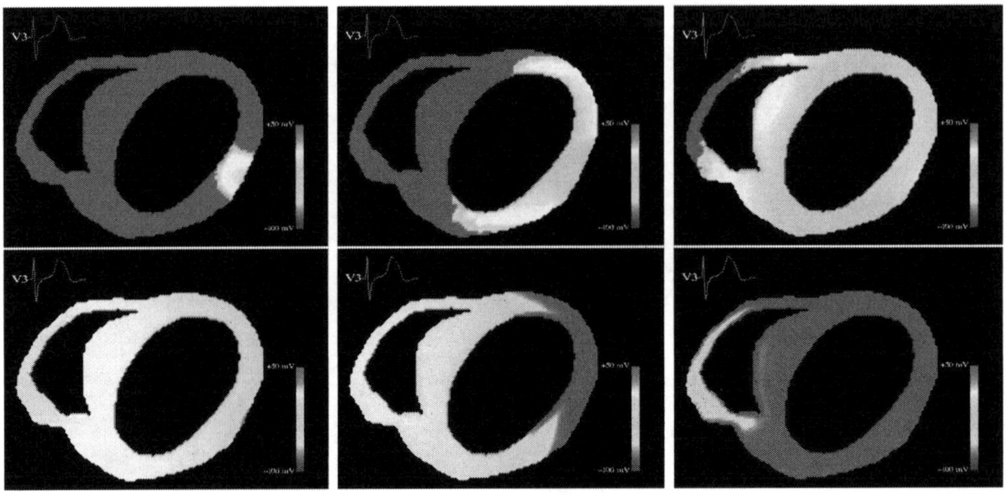

Figure 7.10: *Distributions of transmembrane voltages in the heart during an extrasystolic heart beat: depolarization phase (top), repolarization phase (bottom).*

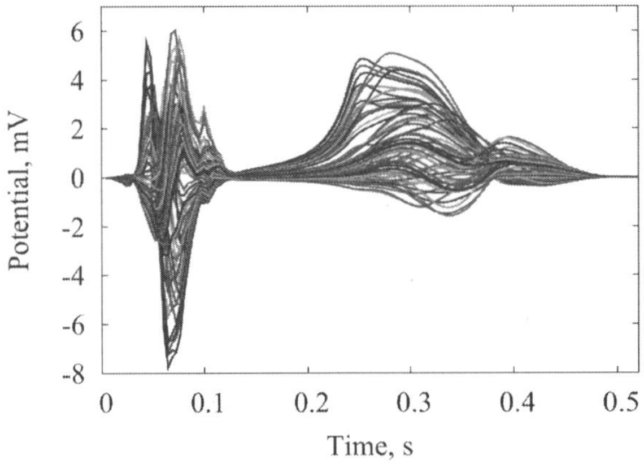

Figure 7.11: *64 channels of simulated ECG for an extrasystolic heart beat.*

7.5 Optimization of the Cardiac Model

The optimization of the cardiac model was performed in two steps: first, the depolarization sequence was varied in order to obtain the best possible QRS-complex, and then the ST-interval was adapted to reconstruct the repolarization phase. The parameters varied in each of these steps are listed in chapter 3.

The comparison between the measured and simulated ECG was done as follows:

1. Both data sets were normalized so that the difference between the maximal and minimal values is 1.

2. The simulated ECG was interpolated to the sample rate of the measured one and shifted so that the R-pikes were aligned.

3. RMS was computed for the difference between the measured and simulated signals for each channel on a predefined time interval (QRS-complex and/or ST-interval).

4. The resulting RMS were averaged.

The resulting value representing the average RMS of the difference of signals in each ECG channel is used as the criterion for optimization. Powell and downhill simplex optimization methods were implemented [150].

Chapter 8

Simulation Results

8.1 Role of Midmyocardial Cells in Forming the ECG

One of the first tasks to be considered using the presented modeling was to investigate the influence of the midmyocardial cells (see Chapter 2) on the resulting ECG. According to [34], the ECG is fully defined by the distributions of TMV on the epi- and endocardial surfaces, if the intracellular and extracellular anisotropy ratios (see Section 4.2) are equal. This fact can significantly decrease the complexity of forward and inverse calculations. The equivalent surface source model is widely used to solve the inverse problem of electrocardiology in terms of ventricular activation times [32, 120].

However according to the recent measurements and simulation studies the anisotropy ratios in intra- and extracellular spaces significantly differ [35, 157]. This fact can cause a major change of the reconstruction results [158]. Therefore the present investigation was aiming to reveal the biases imposed by the assumption of equal anisotropy ratios.

8.1.1 Shifting the M-Cells towards Epi- and Endocardium

The first virtual experiment to unmask the impact of M-cells on the ECG consisted in a shift of the M-cells towards the endo- or epicardium. The way this offset was implemented is shown in figure 8.1. The action potential curves on the surface of the heart were changed only marginally, due to the relatively small resolution of the heart model. Thus one could expect, that in the case of equal anisotropy ratios (or in the case of isotropic ventricular muscle) the changes of the resulting ECG should be negligible.

The ECGs simulated with equal as well as unequal anisotropy ratios are shown in figure 8.2. The changes of the simulated ECG caused by the offset of the M-cells towards endo- and epicardium are shown in figure 8.3.

Although the amplitudes of the both ECGs differ by approximately 25%, the change of ECG caused by the M-cells offset in the case of equal anisotropy ratio (which is caused solely by the modeling errors) is about 10 times smaller than that for unequal anisotropy ratio. This indicates that the M-cells do significantly contribute to the form of ECG in the case of unequal anisotropy ratio.

Since the change in action potential that was applied in this experiment has a large impact on the dispersion of the APD the largest modification of ECG can be observed during the T-wave.

8.1.2 Action Potential Suppression in the M-Cells

Another virtual experiment for the investigation of the contribution of M-cells to the ECG was to suppress the amplitude of action potential in the M-cells by 50%, while leaving that in endo- and epicardial area without changes (see figure 8.4).

The cellular automaton was run with these sets of action potential curves. The simulated ECG was "recorded" and compared for the case of equal as well as unequal anisotropy ratios. The changes of ECG in both cases are shown in figure 8.5

The comparison between the changes of ECG for equal and unequal anisotropy ratios again indicates a significant influence of the M-cells on the resulting ECG.

Since the overall situation after "switching off" the M-cells resembles an infarction in the middle of the ventricular wall, a shift of the ST-segment can be observed.

8.1.3 BSPM Corresponding to the Excited M-Cells

The last experiment allowing to determine the contribution of M-cells to the ECG consisted in the generation of an artificial distribution of TMV within the heart with the following characteristics. A binary erosion filter [159] was applied to the region of the model containing the ventricular myocardium. TMV in the voxels belonging to the remains of myocardium was set to +20 mV ("depolarized"), the voxels where the myocardium had vanished obtained the TMV of -80 mV ("repolarized"). In this way, the whole heart surface remained at rest, with the whole excitation concentrated in the midmyocardial area (figure 8.6).

The forward problem of electrocardiography was solved for such a configuration. In agreement with [34], in the case of equal anisotropy ratios the resulting signal on the surface of the thorax did not exceed $10^{-12}\ mV$. If the anisotropy ratios of intra- and extracellular spaces were different, a BSPM with an amplitude of $2\ mV$ was recorded (figure 8.7).

The latter distribution of TMV can be compared with the physiological situation at the end of the T-wave. Thus the last result indicates, that the form of the T-wave is strongly influenced by the sources located in the midmyocardial area. Ignoring that fact might lead to incorrect results of reconstruction of repolarization times. The results of this investigation were presented in [36].

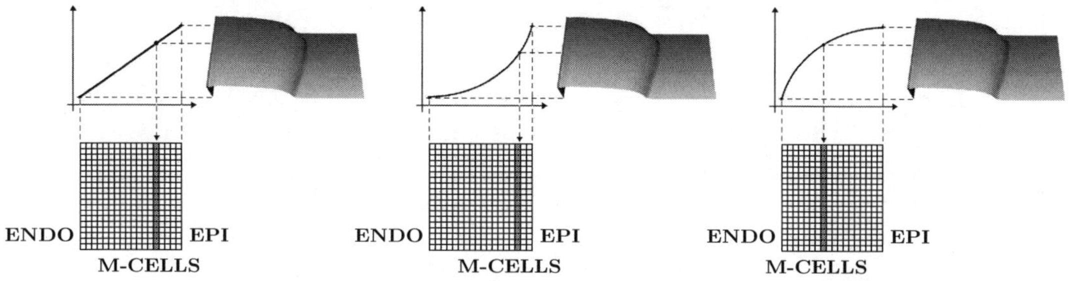

Figure 8.1: *Correspondence between the voxels of the anatomical heart model and the AP-curves: normal transmural dispersion (left); with M-cells shifted towards endocardium (center); towards epicardium (right).*

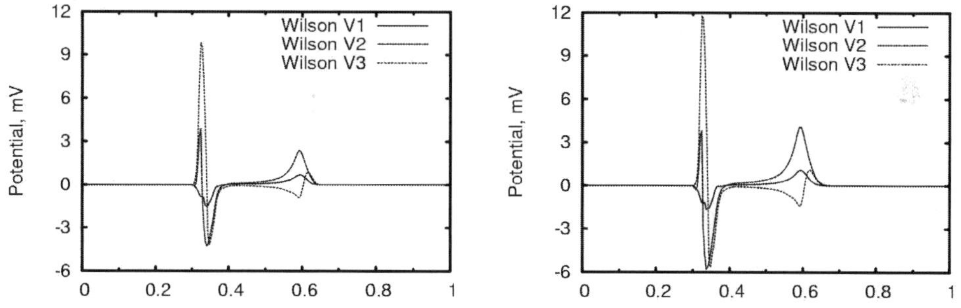

Figure 8.2: *ECGs simulated for the case of equal anisotropy ratio (left) and unequal anisotropy ratio (right) with normal transmural dispersion of action potentials. Wilson leads V1, V2 and V3 are shown.*

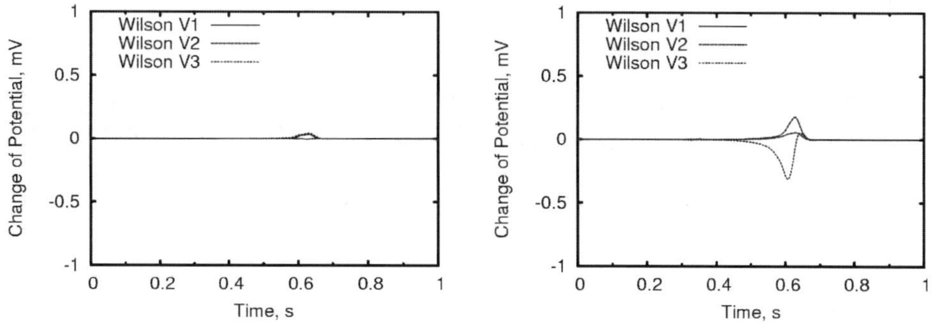

Figure 8.3: *The change of the simulated Wilson leads V1, V2 and V3 resulting from the shift of the M-cells towards epicardium: for the case of equal anisotropy ratio (left), for the case of unequal anisotropy ratio (right).*

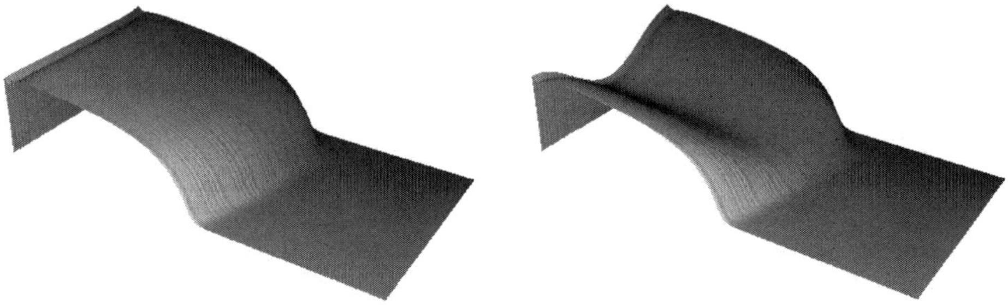

Figure 8.4: *97 action potential curves – original form (left), with M-cells suppressed by 50% (right).*

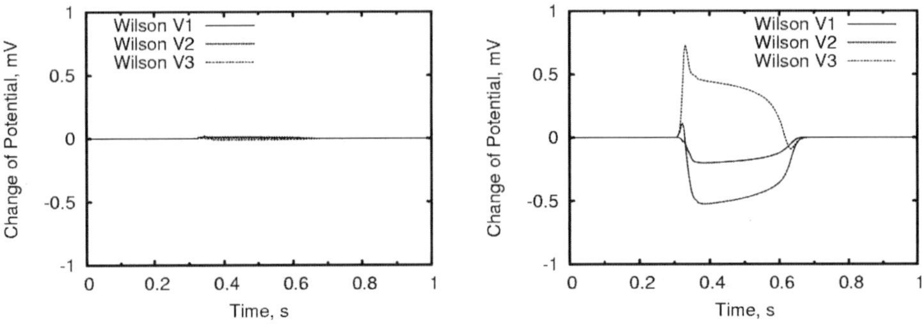

Figure 8.5: *The change of the simulated Wilson leads V1, V2 and V3 resulting from the suppression of action potential amplitude in M-cells by 50% for the case of equal anisotropy ratio (left) and for the case of unequal anisotropy ratio (right).*

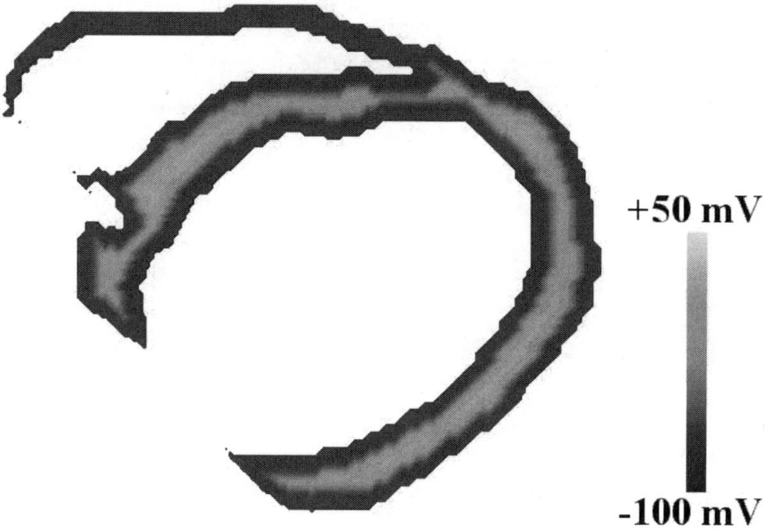

Figure 8.6: *Artificially created distribution of TMV within the ventricular myocardium. The surface of the heart is at rest, whereas the midmyocardial voxels are excited.*

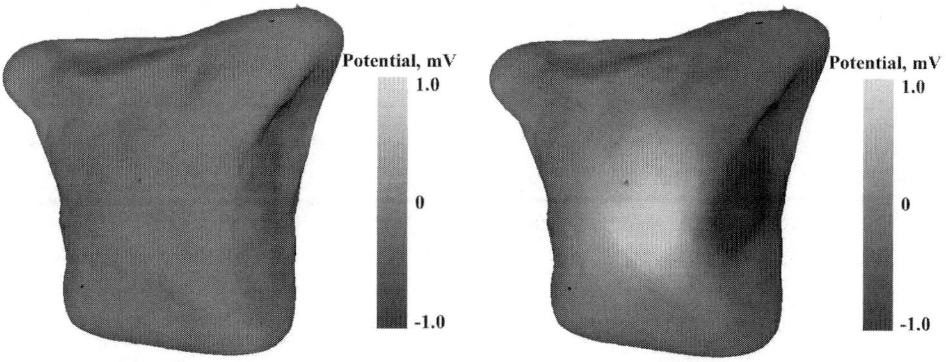

Figure 8.7: *BSPMs corresponding to the distribution of TMV shown in figure 8.6: computed with equal anisotropy ratios (left); with unequal anisotropy ratios (right).*

8.2 Optimization of Depolarization Times

8.2.1 Healthy Subject

The data set of the test subject (see section 6.1) was employed for this investigation. The cardiac and thoracic MRI scans were segmented using deformable triangle meshes. The resulting cardiac model has been shown in figure 7.1. This model has the resolution of $0.5 \times 0.5 \times 0.5\ mm^3$.

The excitation frequency of the heart model is 1 Hz, which is close to the measured data. The cellular automaton was set to a time step of 0.1 ms. The TMV distributions were saved with a time step of 4 ms, thus each heart cycle contained 250 distributions. The modeling of a single heart beat together with the computation of simulated ECG lasted about 30 min. on an Apple XServe with two processors PowerPC G5 2GHz and 2 GB RAM.

Optimized were 6 parameters listed in table 8.1. After a short exploration of the way different parameters were affecting the simulated ECG, the "best" initial values of these parameters were chosen. The ECGSim software [33] was also quite helpful by providing a reference depolarization sequence. After the initial values had been set, 101 optimization steps were performed. The overall optimization time was about 44 hours.

Table 8.1 shows the initial and optimized parameter values. It should be noted, that the values do not necessarily correspond to the reality. There might be other sets of 6 parameters that lead to a low or even lower root-mean-square error. A full search through the 6-dimensional parameter space is not possible. The main function of these parameters is mainly to define the excitation propagation sequence.

Considering the values in table 8.1, it is interesting to note, that the excitation conduction velocity of right ventricular myocardium is large, even larger than that of Purkinje fibers. As the right ventricular wall is relatively thin, it does not matter for the model, if the excitation is conducted rapidly through the right Purkinje fibers and than relatively slowly through the myocardium, or immediately through the myocardium. Other values are quite close to those used e.g. in [52].

The distribution of activation times on the surface of the heart is shown in figure 8.8. The excitation of epicardial surface takes place during 30 ms, the endocardial surface is excited earlier.

The Wilson leads V1 till V5 of measured vs. simulated ECG are compared in figure 8.9.

The distributions of transmembrane voltages and epicardial potentials on the surface of the heart during the depolarization phase as well as corresponding BSPMs are shown in figure 8.10.

8.2.2 Patients with Infarction

The location and extent of an infarction scar were optimized for three patients. QRS-complex and ST-segment were chosen for the computation of optimization criterion (see

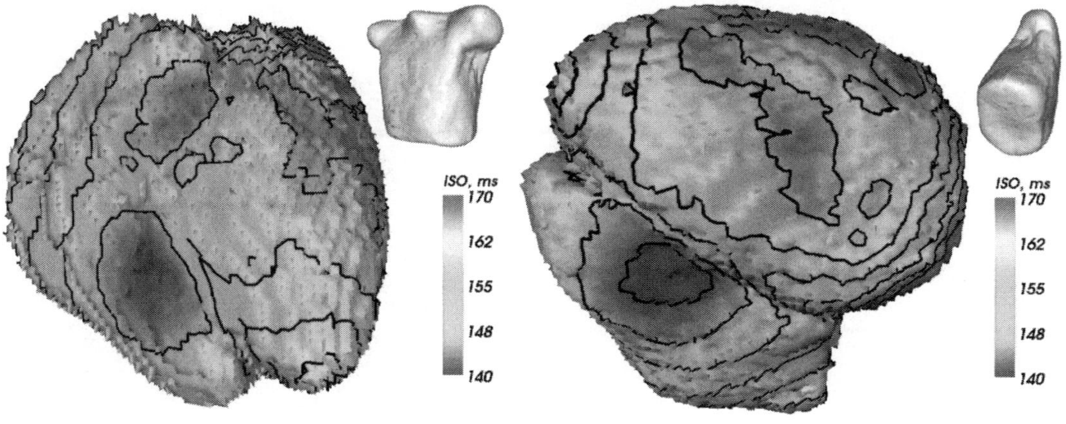

Figure 8.8: *Activation times reconstructed using the optimization-based approach: anterior view (left), posterolateral view (right).*

Tissue Class	Start-up ECV, mm/s	Optimized ECV, mm/s
Left ventricular myocardium	745.502/331.467	979.779/435.632
Right ventricular myocardium	2130.01/947.049	2428.53/1079.78
Right Tawara branch	1574.45	1035.12
Left anterior fascicle	1812.28	1152.38
Right Purkinje fibers	2917.21	2268.99
Left Purkinje fibers	2626.95	3672.73
Root-mean-square	0.1612	0.1126

Table 8.1: *Initial and optimized values of excitation conduction velocity (ECV) in different tissues of a healthy heart. For the tissues with anisotropic ECV longitudinal and transversal values are given. The last line shows the RMS of the difference between simulated and measured ECGs before and after the optimization.*

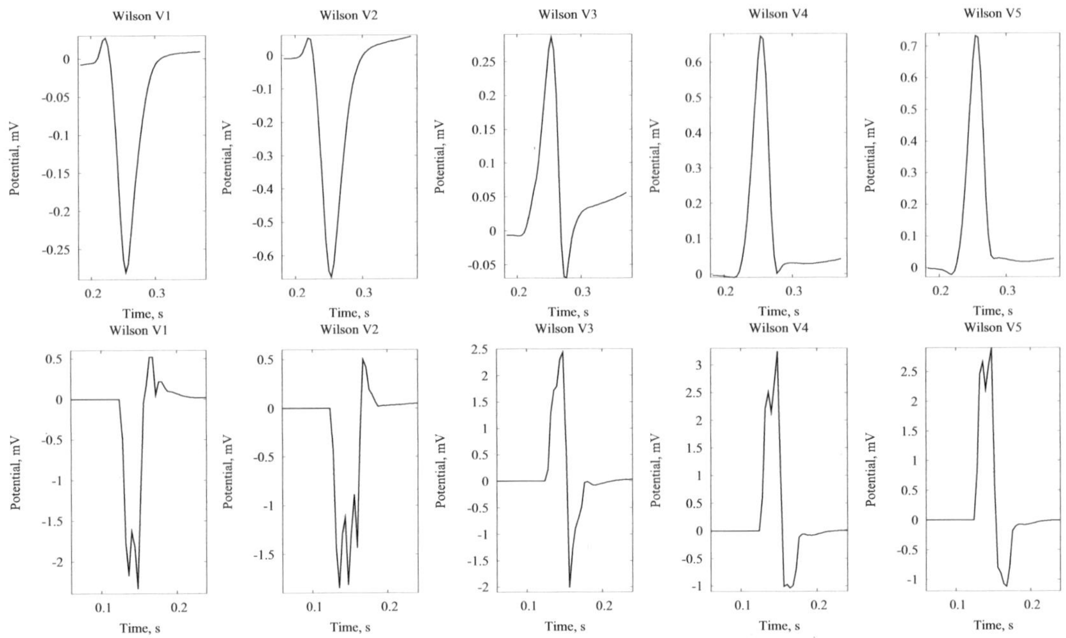

***Figure 8.9:** Wilson leads V1-V5 of the ECG of the healthy person: measured (top) and simulated (bottom).*

figure 8.11).

Two of these patients were considered within the scope of the PhysioNet/Computers in Cardiology Challenge 2007 [160]. The task was to estimate the site and size of an infarction scar from given BSPMs of patients measured in 352 locations.

Since no full 3D data set of the anatomy of the patients was available, in this case the MEETMan data set was employed to reproduce the patient's anatomy. The triangle mesh with electrodes at its nodes was manually deformed to fit the surface of the thorax. Afterwards the electrodes were projected onto the surface of the volume conductor (see figure 8.12).

The measured vs. simulated Wilson leads V1-V5 of the first patient ("case 3") are shown in figure 8.14. The simulated V_1 lead shows a wrong Q-wave, which was not observed during the measurement. Still the rest of the leads – mainly those related to the left ventricle – show a good correspondence between measurement and simulation.

The infarction scar found for the first patient is shown in figure 8.13. The infarction is located in the lateral wall, with the center in the 12th AHA segment. It covers about 10% of the ventricular myocardium.

Figure 8.15 depicts the location of the infarction scar found for the second patient ("case 4") of the Challenge. This infarction covers only 0.2% of the ventricular myocardium. Measured and simulated ECG of the patient 4 are compared in figure 8.16.

The discrepancies between the obtained results and the real values are shown in table 8.2.

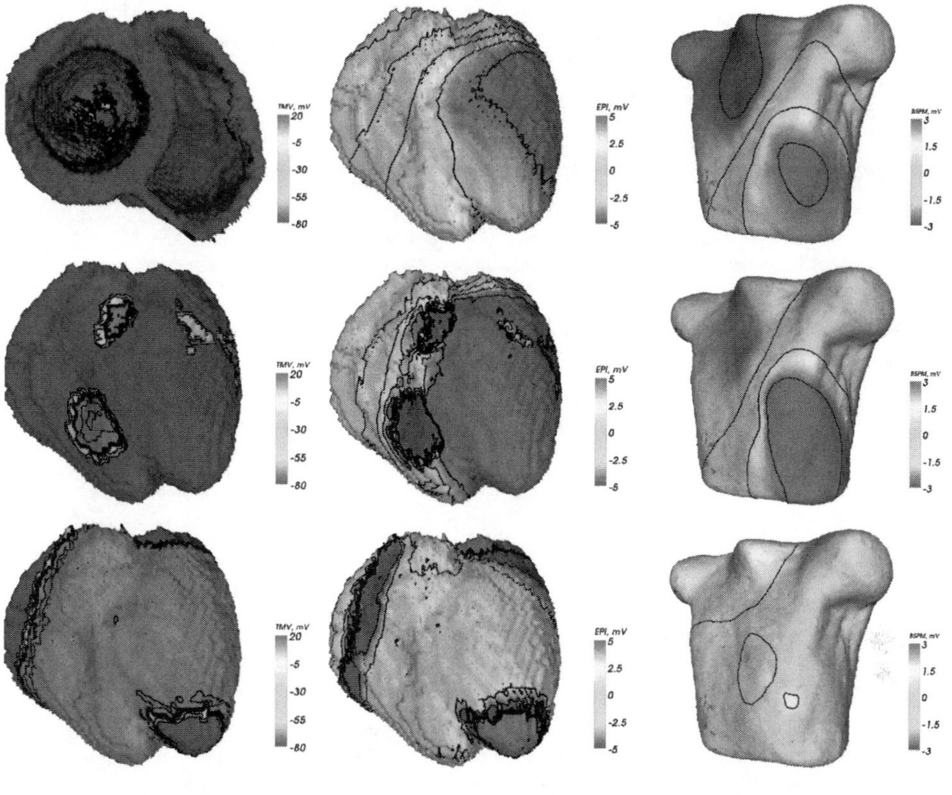

Figure 8.10: *Simulated distributions of transmembrane voltages (left), epicardial potentials (center) and body surface potentials (right) for 3 time instants during the QRS-complex. Simulation was performed for the healthy subject.*

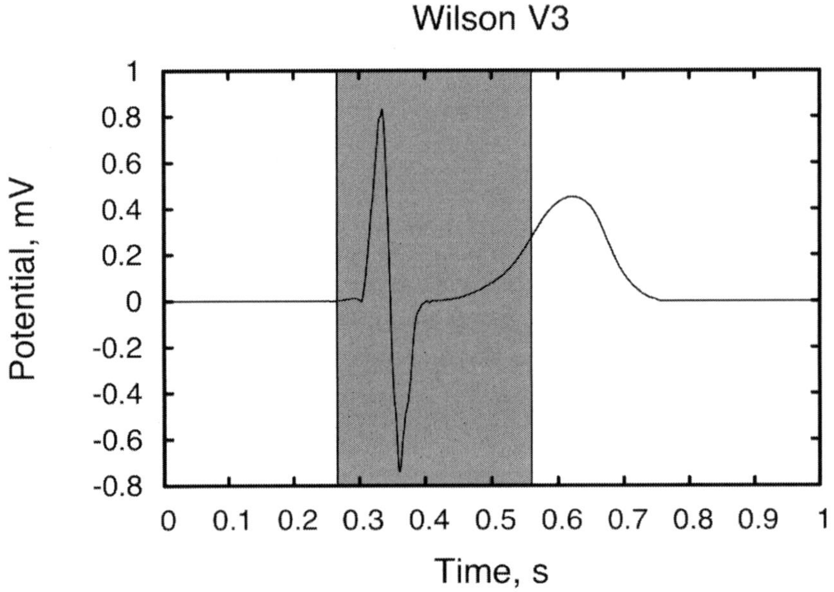

Figure 8.11: *Wilson lead V3 of a patient with infarction. The range considered for the optimization of infarction location and extent is selected.*

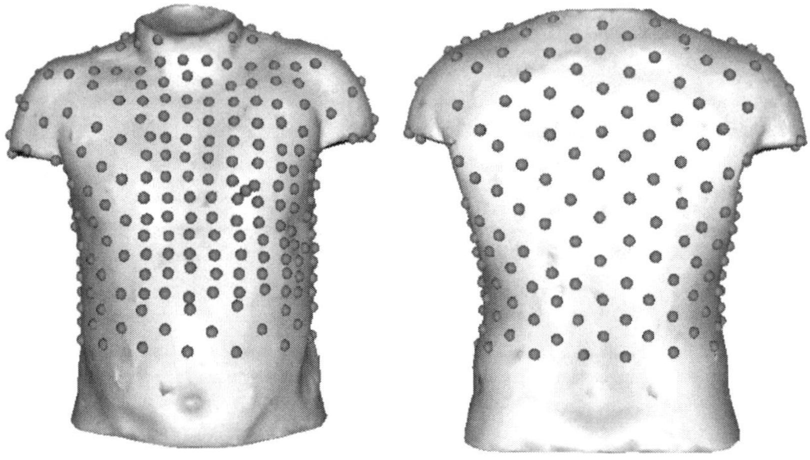

Figure 8.12: *352 sites of BSPM recording used for the reconstruction of infarction scar in scope of PhysioNet/Computers in Cardiology Challenge 2007.*

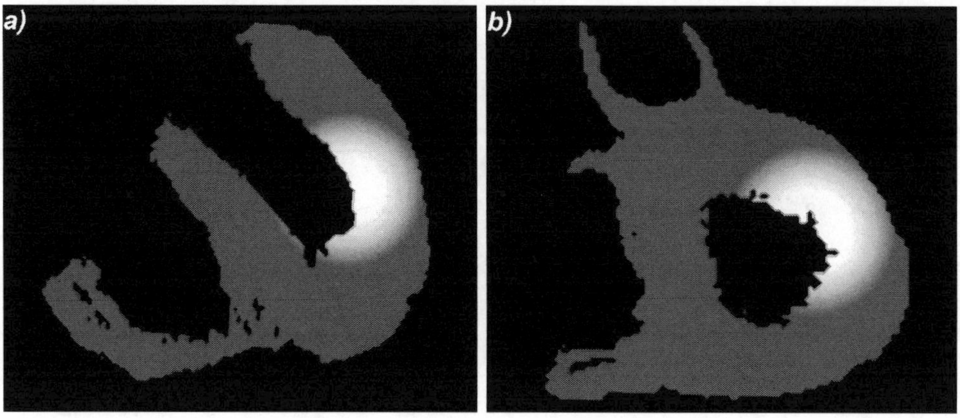

Figure 8.13: *Infarcted area found for the first patient of the PhysioNet Challenge. Transverse (a) and frontal (b) slices are shown. Infarcted tissue is shown with white color.*

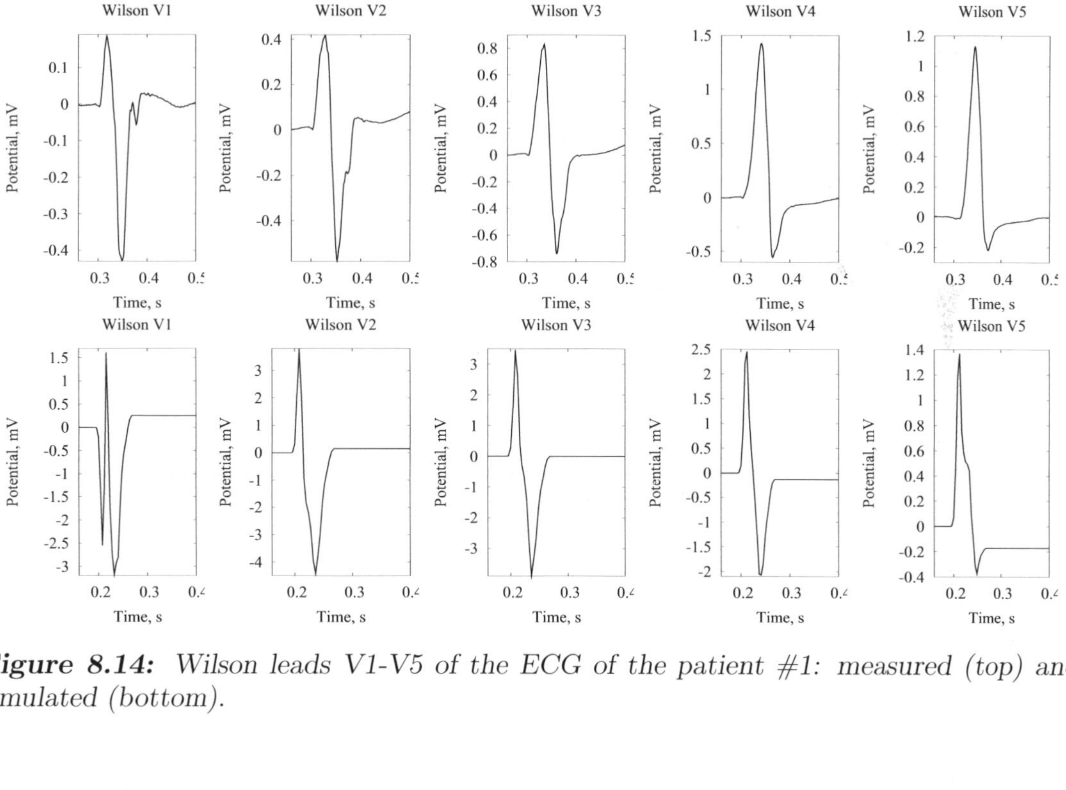

Figure 8.14: *Wilson leads V1-V5 of the ECG of the patient #1: measured (top) and simulated (bottom).*

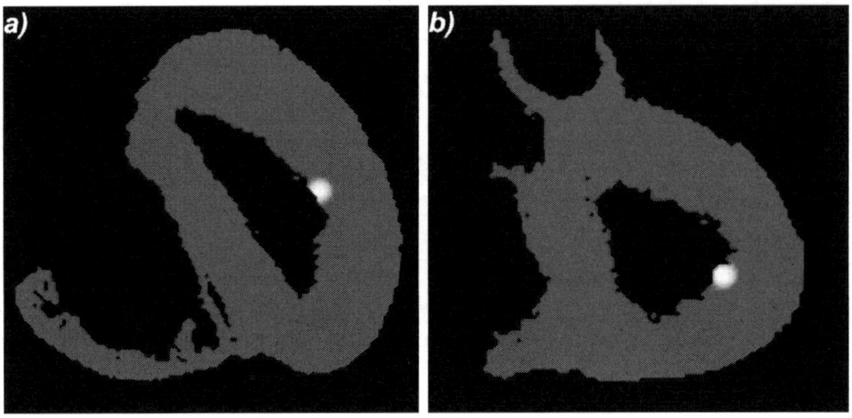

Figure 8.15: *Infarcted area found for the second patient of the PhysioNet Challenge. Colors and views correspond to those in figure 8.13.*

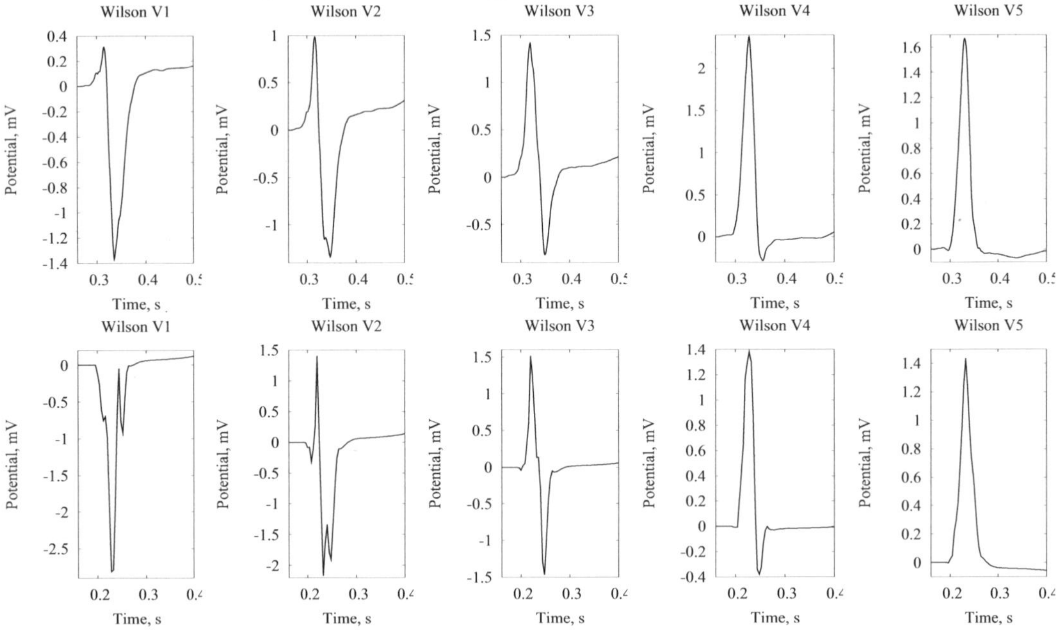

Figure 8.16: *Wilson leads V1-V5 of the ECG of the patient #2: measured (top) and simulated (bottom).*

	Case 3	Case 4
EPD	43	14
SO	0.400	0.167
CED	1	1

Table 8.2: *Discrepancies between the estimation of the infarction site and size made in this paper and the real values. EPD: the percentage discrepancy of the extent of infarctions; SO: the overlap between the sets of segments affected by infarction (0-1, 1 is the perfect match); CED: the distance between the centroids of estimated and real infarctions (0-4, 0 is the perfect match).*

The localization error for each infarction did not exceed 1 AHA segment in each case. Still the error of the size estimation was quite large (see table 8.2). The following reasons might cause such an effect:

- The patient might suffer from ischemia instead of infarction;
- The assumption of a spherical infarction scar might be wrong;
- Other modeling errors might affect the quality of solution, such as errors in body geometry, conductivity values etc.

Another problem encountered during the solution consists in a large amount of local minima of the optimization criterion in the space of model parameters. Several different values of parameters might lead to very similar modeling results. At least 3 different sets of initial values were used for each patient in order to find the global minimum.

Concluding this investigation, the presented way to optimize the site and size of infarction scar is able to deliver the correct location, although the estimation of size has failed. Still this optimization is not supposed to be used in clinical practice: the aim of the research was just to prove the correctness of infarction simulation. The location of infarction can be found from the solution of the inverse problem (see chapters 5 and 9), or from MRI data sets with introduced contrast agent in order to be built into the electrophysiological model of the patient's heart. Such a model can be a useful tool for cardiologists helping to investigate the individual anomalies of de- and repolarization of patient's heart and to estimate the stability of the heart function.

The results shown in this subsection were presented in [161].

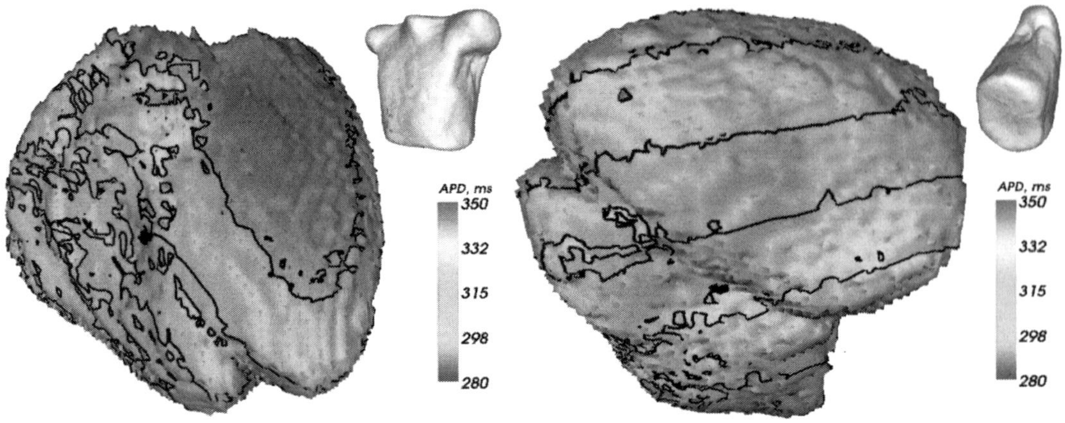

Figure 8.17: *Distribution of action potential duration resulting from the optimization of APD gradient for a healthy heart. Transmural dispersion was kept constant. Anterior view (left) and posterolateral view (right) are shown.*

8.3 T-wave of a Healthy Subject

The optimization of repolarizaton sequence for a healthy heart was performed using the data set of the healthy subject (see section 6.1). The form of the simulated QRS-complex had been previously optimized as described in section 8.2.

The form of the T-wave was optimized in two steps. First, a gradient of action potential duration (APD) was introduced, its size (that is, the change of APD per 1 mm), direction as well of the size of APD in the center of the left ventricle were optimized (see section 7.3). The transmural dispersion of APD was kept constant as determined by ten Tusscher cell model [22] (see section 7.3, figure 7.3).

Figure 8.17 depicts the distribution of action potential duration on the surface of the heart for this case. APD varies within the range between 280 (left ventricle anterior) and 350 (right ventricle posterobasal) ms.

Simulated Wilson leads V1-V5 resulting from the optimization of APD gradient are shown in figure 8.18 (right). They can be compared with the measured ECG leads shown in the same figure, left.

Three distributions of transmembrane voltage, epicardial potential and body surface potential during the T-wave are shown in figure 8.19. The repolarization starts on the anterior wall of the left ventricle. The software package ECGSim [33] delivers quite similar results. Also the solutions of inverse problem show the same feature (see chapter 9).

The optimization of transmural APD dispersion did not result in major modifications of the APD distribution. The result of this optimization is shown in figure 8.20. Figure 8.21 contains the Wilson V1-V5 leads simulated with the optimal parameters of APD distribution (right) compared with measured data (left). The simulated distributions of TMV, epicardial potentials and BSPMs at the beginning, in the middle and at the end of the T-wave are shown in figure 8.22.

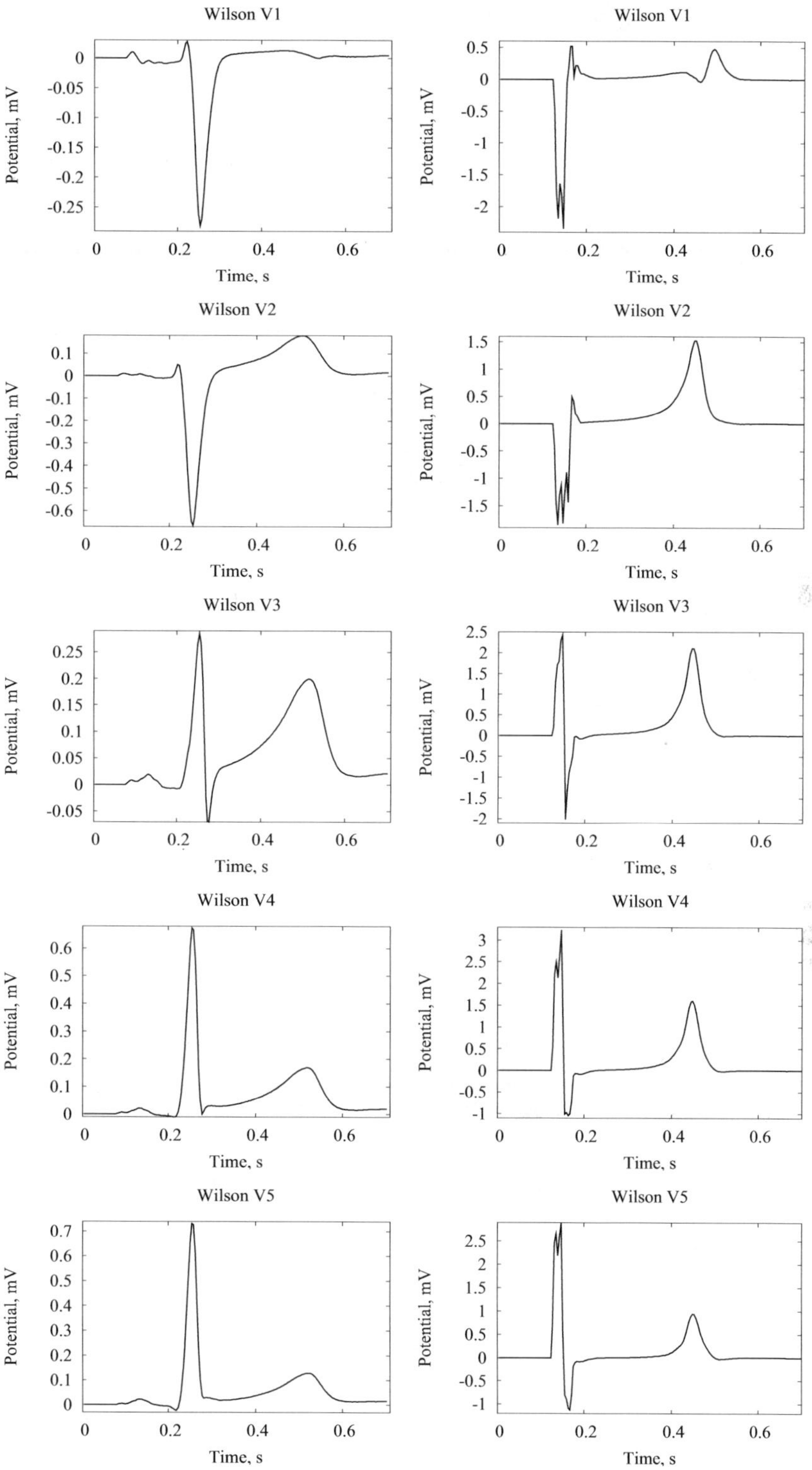

Figure 8.18: *Wilson leads V1-V5 of the ECG of the healthy person: measured (left) and simulated (right). The gradient of APD was optimized in order to obtain a better T-wave.*

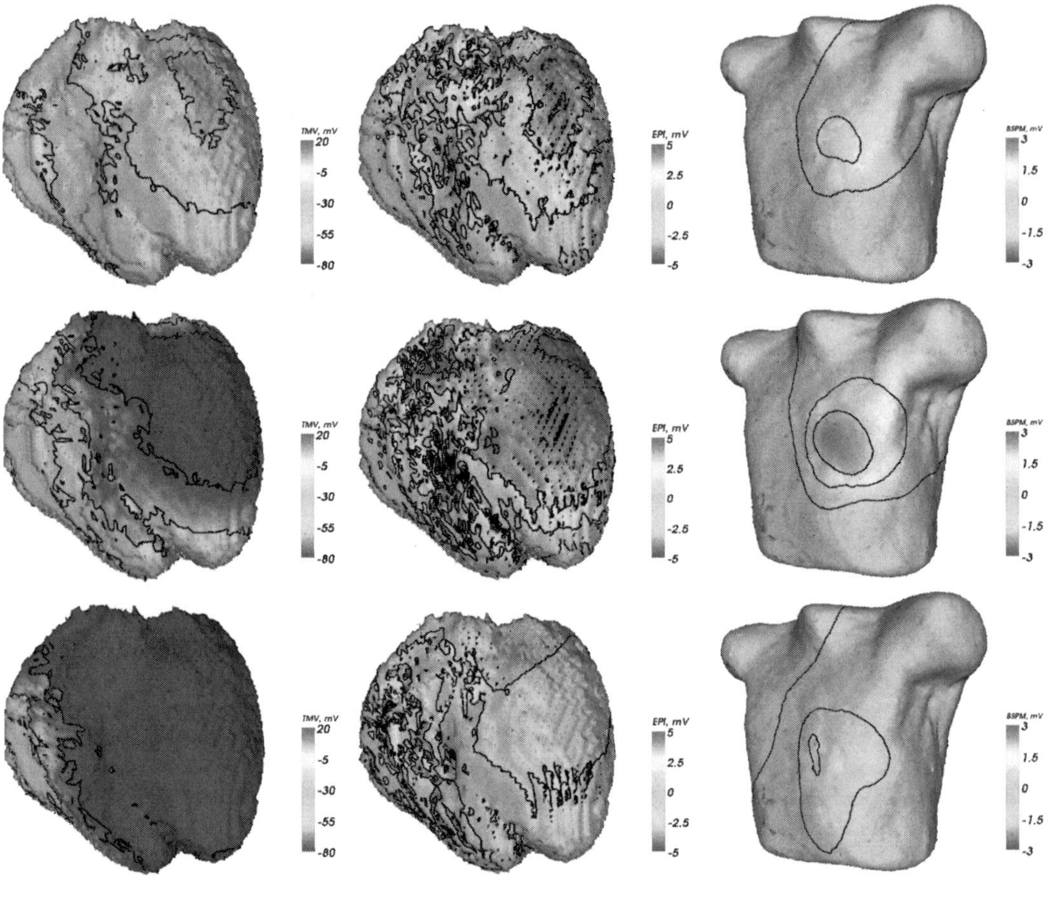

Figure 8.19: *Simulated distributions of transmembrane voltages (left), epicardial potentials (center) and body surface potentials (right) for 3 time instants during the T-wave. Simulation was performed for the healthy subject. The repolarization sequence was modified by optimization of the APD gradient, the transmural dispersion of APD was kept constant.*

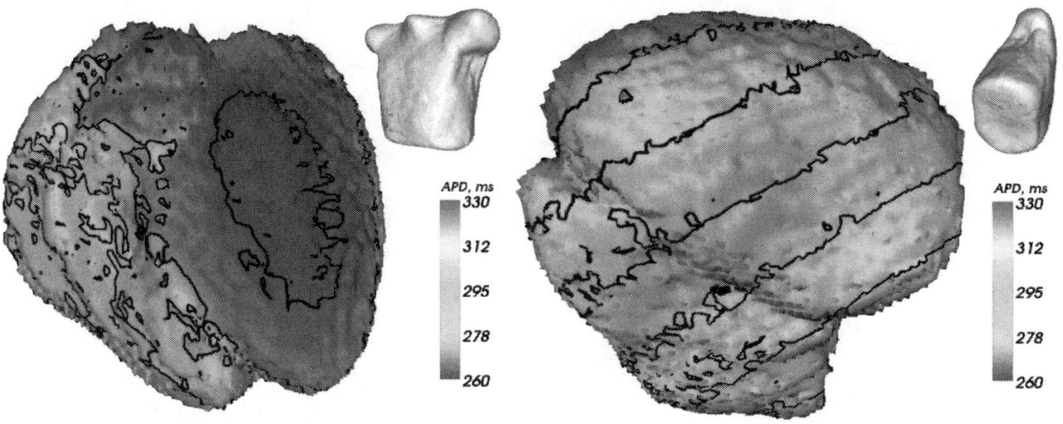

Figure 8.20: *Distribution of action potential duration resulting from the optimization of APD gradient as well as the transmural dispersion of APD for a healthy heart. Anterior view (left) and posterolateral view (right) are shown.*

Parameter Name	1st optimization	2nd optimization
APD, endocardium	317 ms	289 ms
APD, M-cells	360 ms	321 ms
APD, epicardium	306 ms	280 ms
APD gradient, azimuth	65.6^o	72.7^o
APD gradient, declination	106.0^o	118.5^o
APD gradient, size ($ms \cdot mm^{-1}$)	0.00251	0.00259

Table 8.3: *The parameters of APD dispersion after the 1st optimization step, consisting in the optimization of APD gradient only, and after the 2nd optimization step, where both APD gradient and transmural APD dispersion were optimized.*

The parameters of APD distributions resulting from both steps of optimization with their optimized values are listed in table 8.3. The orientation of APD gradient has not changed significantly after the second optimization step; both approaches show the repolarization of the left anterior ventricular wall first. Reconstructions in [33] also show an earlier repolarization in the right ventricle, which could not be described by a linear approximation of APD dispersion. Still the simulated BSPMs during the T-wave strongly resemble the measured ones (see figure 9.10 in chapter 9). Thus it can be concluded that at least qualitatively a correct distribution of APD within a healthy heart has been achieved.

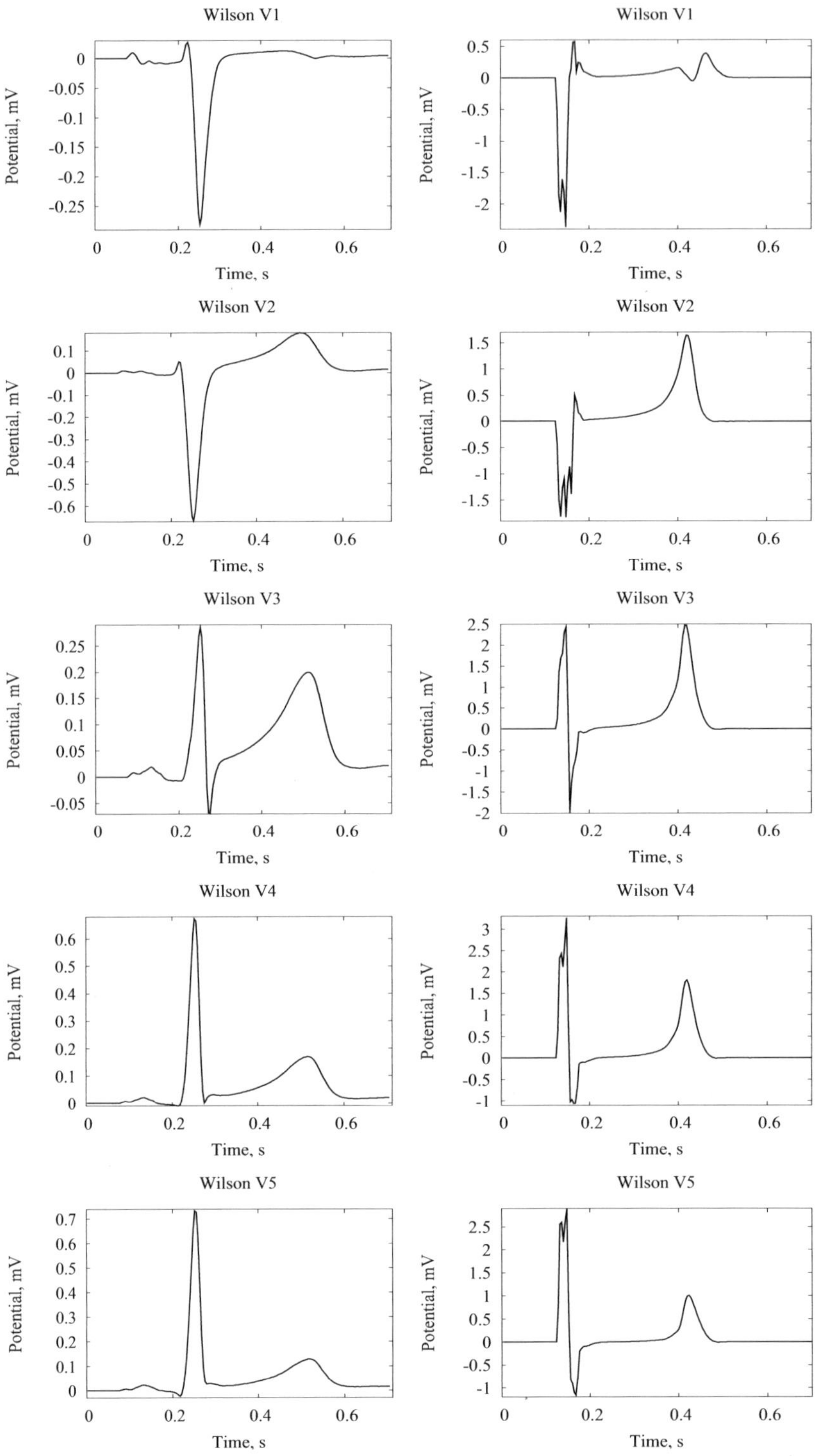

Figure 8.21: *Wilson leads V1-V5 of the ECG of the healthy person: measured (left) and simulated (right). The gradient of APD and transmural APD dispersion were optimized in order to obtain a better T-wave.*

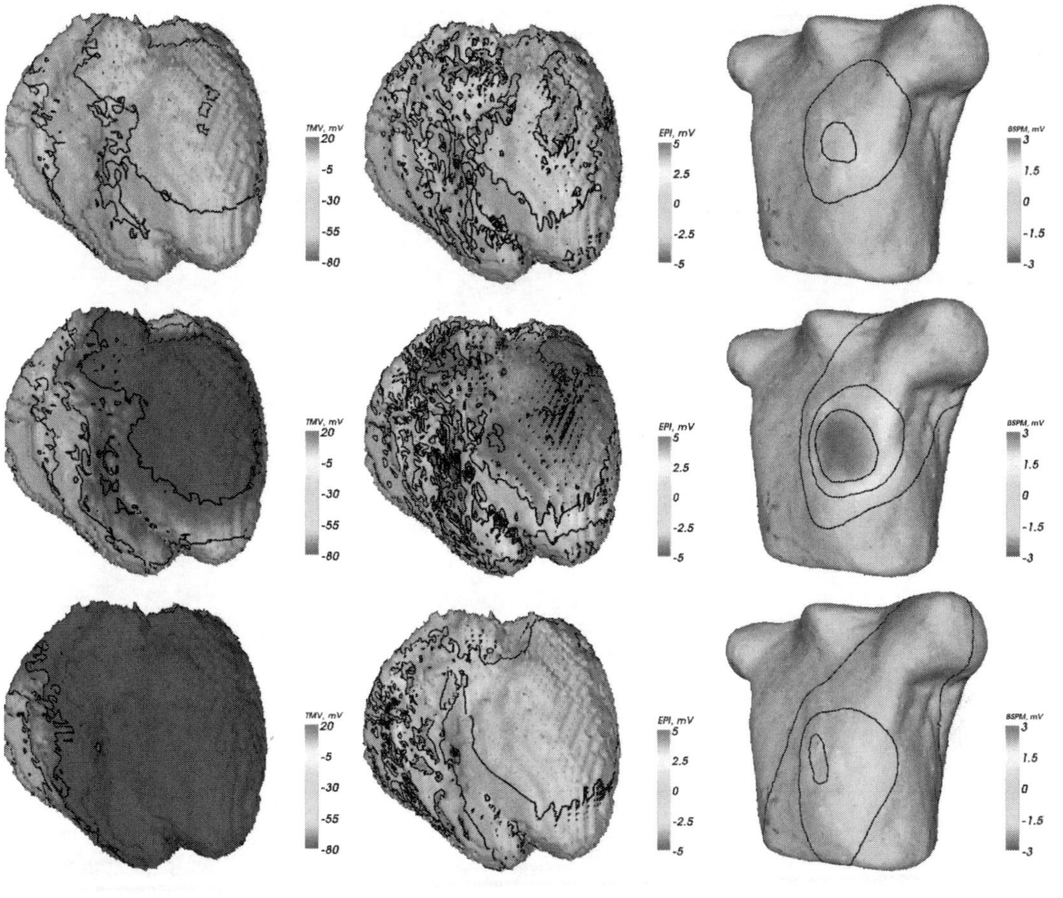

Figure 8.22: *Simulated distributions of transmembrane voltages (left), epicardial potentials (center) and body surface potentials (right) for 3 time instants during the T-wave. Simulation was performed for the healthy subject. The repolarization sequence was modified by optimization of the APD gradient and transmural APD dispersion.*

8.4 Change of ECG Caused by Infarction

8.4.1 Introduction

It is well known that the ischemic disease is the main cause of the ST-segment shift in ECG. The character of this shift depends on different factors: the site and size of ischemic region, the stage of disorder, physical activity of the patient etc. Several research groups consider the dependence of ST-segment morphology on the geometry of the affected area [162, 163, 164, 165, 166].

In [164] the ischemic region consisted of 3 concentric areas with mild, moderate and severe ischemia. These tissues possessed different action potential curves, with APD decreasing and onset duration increasing with the severity of ischemia. The closure of left anterior descending, left circumflex and right coronary arteries was considered. The size of the ischemic region was not varied.

In [166] only the ST segment shifts were considered for minor subendocardial infarctions. The change of the QRS complex was not considered.

8.4.2 Description of Simulation

In the current work 90 infarction scars surrounded with ischemic tissue are considered. This set includes 10 different infarction locations: 1 apical, 4 around the apex and 5 basal. These locations are shown in figure 8.23. As the heart is shown in different orientations in order to show the infarction, the corresponding thorax view is displayed next to each image.

Also 3 different sizes of infarction scar are considered, with diameters equal to 20, 30 and 50 *mm*. Three lateral infarctions (location 3) with these sizes are displayed in figure 8.24. In this figure a transverse cross-section of the heart is shown.

The third parameter being varied in this set of infarctions is the transmural location (or "depth") of infarction. This variation is shown in figure 8.25. Again, three lateral infarctions with the diameter of 30 *mm* are shown. In the left image ("case 0") endocardium is affected most. The central image corresponds to a transmural infarction, the center of ischemic area is located in the middle of the ventricle wall ("case 1"). The right image represents the quite unusual – but still possible [15] – case of epicardial infarction ("case 2").

The whole set of infarctions is indexed according to these parameters. In these 3-digit indices the first digit denotes the location of infarction scar (as in figure 8.23). The second digit represents the size of the ischemic area (see figure 8.24). Finally, the third digit corresponds to the transmural location ("depth") of infarction (figure 8.24).

In this notation figure 8.23 demonstrates the infarctions with indices 021, 121, ..., 921. In figure 8.24 cases 301, 311, 321 are displayed. Finally, cases 310, 311 and 312 are shown in figure 8.25.

In order to improve the quality of simulations, the data set of the test subject has been employed. Excitation conduction velocities of various tissue classes as well as the APD dispersion within the myocardium have previously been optimized as shown in sections 8.2

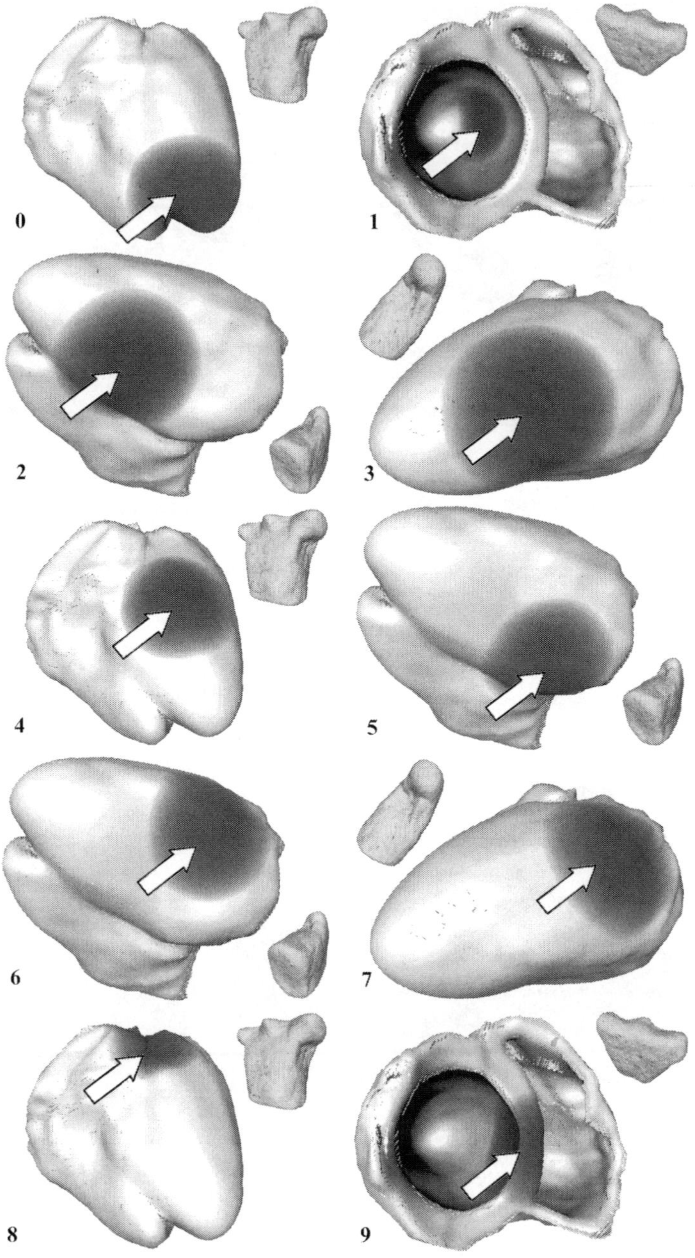

Figure 8.23: *Locations of simulated infarction scar used in table 8.4. The number in the lower left corner of each image corresponds to the first digit of infarction index in the table.*

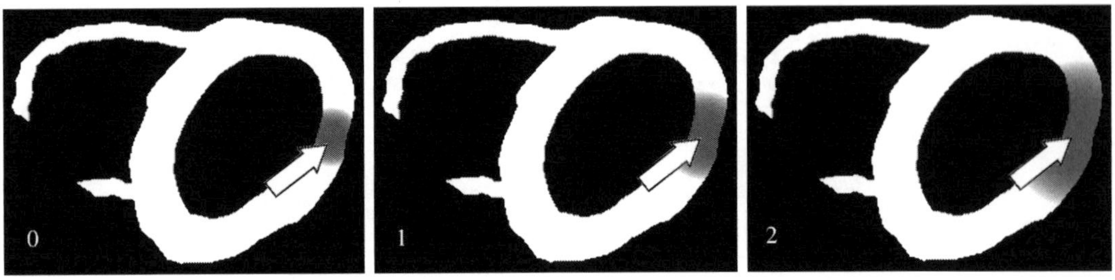

Figure 8.24: *Sizes of simulated infarction scar used in table 8.4. The number in the lower left corner of each image corresponds to the second digit of infarction index in the table.*

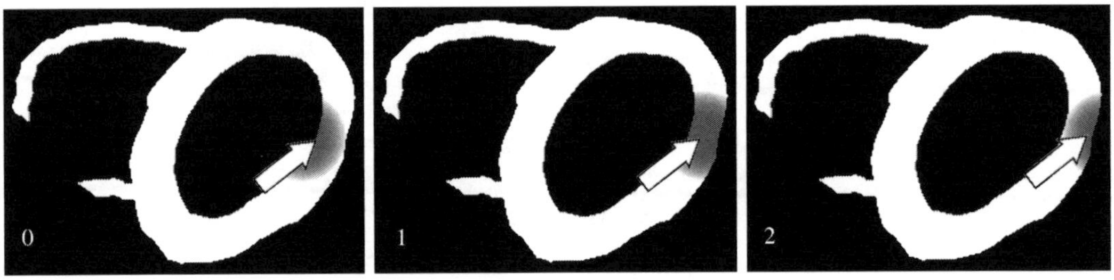

Figure 8.25: *Depths of simulated infarction scar (endo-, M- and epicardial locations) used in table 8.4. The number in the lower left corner of each image corresponds to the third digit of infarction index in the table.*

and 8.3. For each simulation step an infarction with predefined parameters is introduced and the corresponding "pathological" ECG is computed, from which the "healthy" ECG can be subtracted in order to obtain the infarction-related changes.

8.4.3 Simulation Results

The following figures demonstrate the changes of cardiac electrophysiology caused by anterior infarctions. The influence of a transmural anterior infarction (index 421) on the distributions of epicardial and body surface potentials is illustrated in figure 8.26. The change of multichannel ECG caused by this type of infarction is shown in figure 8.27. Similar features are experimentally observed in the case of patient 4, see section 9.6.

The distributions of transmembrane voltage, epicardial potential and body surface potential during the ST-segment for the case of endocardial anterior infarction (index 410) are shown in figure 8.28. Figure 8.27 demonstrates the changes in the simulated 64-channel ECG.

Table 8.4 sums up the results obtained in the course of simulations. The signals in standard leads during the ST-segment are shown for 91 cases ("healthy" and 90 infarctions). The first column of this table contains the infarction indices as described above. The following 13 columns contain the signal amplitude in leads V1, V2, V3, V4, V5, V6, aVF, aVR, aVL, I, II, III and Wilson Central Terminal (WCT). These signals are caused primarily by the displacement currents flowing through the extracellular space out of the infarcted area (which has a smaller TMV) towards the healthy myocardium.

The following notation is used in table 8.4 for the potential measured in each lead during the ST-segment. First, for each infarction the overall amplitude of simulated ECG (including the QRS-complex and the T-wave) in all 9 channels is found. Afterwards the signal in each lead in the middle of the ST-segment is normalized by this overall amplitude. If the resulting ratio is larger than 5%, which means a strong ST elevation, the (++) sign is put into the corresponding cell of the table. For ratios between 1% and 5% (+) sign is used. If the ratio is between -1% and +1%, 0 is written. In the case of ST-depression, (-) or (- -) signs are used for the small and large depressions, respectively.

The locations of standard electrodes on the test subject's thorax are shown in figure 8.30. These locations have been selected according to [12].

Table 8.4: *Simulated offsets of ST-segment for different infarction locations, sizes and depths. First column displays a 3-digit index. The first digit of this index characterizes the location of infarction (see figure 8.23), second – size (figure 8.24), third – depth (figure 8.25). HLTH denotes the "healthy" case. The rest of columns contain the size of ST-segment offset. (++) stands for the elevation of more than 5% of overall signal amplitude, (+) for over 1%, (0) means a small offset between -1% and +1%, (-) denotes the ST depression of less than 5%, (- -) – more than 5%.*

Index	**V1**	**V2**	**V3**	**V4**	**V5**	**V6**	**aVF**	**aVR**	**aVL**	**I**	**II**	**III**	**WCT**
HLTH	0	0	0	0	0	0	0	0	0	0	0	0	0

Index	V1	V2	V3	V4	V5	V6	aVF	aVR	aVL	I	II	III	WCT
000	+	+	0	-	-	0	-	+	0	0	-	-	0
001	0	+	+	+	0	0	-	0	0	0	-	-	0
002	0	0	+	+	0	0	0	0	0	0	0	0	0
010	+	+	0	-	-	0	- -	+	+	0	- -	- -	+
011	0	+	+	++	+	0	-	0	0	0	0	-	0
012	0	0	+	+	+	0	+	-	0	0	+	+	0
020	+	++	++	++	++	+	- -	+	++	+	- -	- -	++
021	-	0	++	++	++	0	0	-	+	+	+	0	+
022	-	-	+	++	+	0	+	-	-	+	++	+	+
100	0	0	+	0	0	0	0	0	0	0	0	-	0
101	0	0	0	0	0	0	0	0	0	0	0	0	0
102	+	0	-	-	-	0	0	+	0	0	-	0	-
110	0	0	0	+	+	+	-	0	+	+	0	-	+
111	0	0	- -	-	-	0	0	+	0	-	-	0	-
112	+	+	-	-	-	-	0	+	-	-	-	0	-
120	0	-	- -	- -	-	0	-	0	0	0	-	-	+
121	+	0	- -	- -	- -	-	-	+	-	-	-	0	-
122	+	+	- -	- -	- -	-	-	+	-	-	-	+	- -
200	+	+	+	+	0	0	-	+	+	0	-	-	0
201	0	+	+	0	0	0	-	0	0	0	-	-	0
202	0	0	0	0	0	0	0	0	0	0	0	0	0
210	+	+	+	+	0	0	-	+	+	0	-	-	+
211	0	0	0	0	0	0	0	0	0	0	0	-	+
212	-	-	-	-	0	0	+	-	-	0	+	+	0
220	0	+	+	+	+	+	-	0	+	+	-	-	++
221	-	-	0	0	0	0	+	-	0	+	+	+	+
222	-	-	-	-	0	0	++	-	-	+	++	++	+
300	+	+	+	0	-	0	-	+	0	0	-	-	0
301	0	+	0	0	0	0	-	0	0	0	-	-	0
302	0	0	0	0	+	+	0	0	0	0	0	0	0
310	+	+	+	-	-	-	-	+	0	-	-	-	-
311	0	+	0	-	0	+	-	0	0	0	-	-	0
312	-	-	0	0	+	+	+	-	0	+	+	0	0
320	+	+	-	- -	-	0	- -	+	+	-	- -	- -	-
321	0	0	-	-	++	+	0	0	+	0	0	-	0
322	-	-	-	0	++	++	+	-	0	+	+	+	+
400	0	0	-	-	-	0	0	0	0	0	-	0	0
401	0	0	+	+	0	0	-	0	0	0	0	-	0
402	0	0	+	+	0	0	0	0	0	0	0	0	0
410	+	0	-	-	-	-	-	+	0	-	-	0	0
411	0	0	++	++	+	0	-	0	+	+	-	-	0
412	0	0	++	++	+	+	0	0	+	+	0	-	0

Index	V1	V2	V3	V4	V5	V6	aVF	aVR	aVL	I	II	III	WCT
420	0	0	++	++	0	0	-	+	+	0	-	-	+
421	-	+	++	++	++	+	-	0	+	+	-	- -	+
422	-	+	++	++	++	+	-	-	+	+	0	-	+
500	0	+	+	0	0	0	-	0	0	0	-	-	0
501	0	0	+	0	0	0	0	0	0	0	0	-	0
502	0	0	0	0	0	0	0	0	0	0	0	0	0
510	0	+	+	+	0	0	-	0	+	0	-	-	+
511	0	0	0	0	0	0	0	0	0	0	0	0	+
512	0	0	0	0	0	0	0	0	0	0	0	0	0
520	-	0	+	+	+	+	0	-	+	+	0	-	+
521	-	-	0	+	+	+	+	-	0	+	+	0	+
522	-	-	0	0	0	0	0	0	0	0	0	0	+
600	+	+	+	0	0	0	-	+	0	0	-	-	0
601	+	+	+	0	0	0	-	+	0	0	-	-	0
602	0	0	0	0	0	0	0	0	0	0	0	0	0
610	+	+	+	+	0	-	-	+	+	-	- -	-	0
611	0	+	+	0	0	0	0	0	0	0	-	0	0
612	-	0	0	0	0	+	0	-	0	0	+	0	0
620	+	+	+	0	-	-	-	+	0	-	-	-	0
621	0	0	0	0	0	0	0	0	0	0	0	0	0
622	-	0	0	0	0	+	0	0	0	0	+	0	0
700	+	+	0	0	0	0	-	+	0	0	-	0	0
701	0	0	0	0	0	0	-	0	0	0	-	-	0
702	0	0	0	0	0	+	-	0	+	0	0	-	0
710	+	+	0	-	-	-	-	+	0	-	-	-	-
711	0	0	0	0	0	+	-	0	+	0	-	-	0
712	0	0	0	0	+	+	-	0	+	+	-	-	0
720	+	+	-	-	0	+	- -	+	+	0	- -	- -	0
721	0	0	0	0	+	+	- -	+	+	+	-	- -	0
722	0	0	0	+	+	+	-	0	+	+	-	- -	+
800	0	-	-	0	0	0	0	0	0	0	0	0	0
801	0	0	0	0	0	0	0	0	0	0	-	0	0
802	+	+	0	0	0	0	-	+	0	0	-	-	0
810	-	-	-	0	0	0	0	0	0	0	0	0	0
811	0	0	-	-	-	0	-	+	0	0	-	-	0
812	+	+	-	-	-	0	-	+	0	0	-	-	0
820	+	+	0	-	-	-	-	+	+	-	-	-	+
821	+	+	+	-	-	-	-	+	+	-	- -	-	+
822	+	+	0	-	-	-	-	+	+	-	-	-	0
900	0	0	+	0	0	0	0	0	0	0	0	0	0
901	0	0	0	0	0	0	-	0	0	0	-	0	0
902	+	+	0	0	0	0	-	0	0	0	-	0	0

Index	V1	V2	V3	V4	V5	V6	aVF	aVR	aVL	I	II	III	WCT
910	-	0	0	+	0	0	0	0	0	0	0	0	+
911	+	0	0	0	0	0	-	+	0	0	-	-	0
912	+	+	0	0	0	0	-	+	0	-	-	-	-
920	0	-	-	0	0	0	-	0	0	0	-	-	0
921	+	0	-	-	-	0	-	+	0	-	-	-	-
922	+	+	0	-	-	-	-	+	0	-	-	-	-

8.4.4 Conclusions

According to the data listed in table 8.4, there exist two different mechanisms of ST-segment offset. One of them prevails in the case of large transmural infarctions, the other corresponds to the non-Q-wave infarctions.

It follows from the bidomain model, that any infarction independently from its size entails a positively charged area in the ventricular myocardium. Such an area can be seen in figure 8.26, center (infarction index 421). The surrounding tissue has a negative charge. Thus in the case of a large transmural infarction a dipole appears directed towards the infarction site (see figure 8.31). The BSPM reproduces this dipole, which means that there appears an area of positive potential at the side of infarction (see figure 8.26, right). In table 8.4 the infarction with index 421 is characterized by large positive signals in leads V3-V5.

Let us now consider a purely endocardial infarction. The positive area is then located at the endocardium, whereas the epicardium is negatively charged. Therefore although the dipole vector is still oriented towards the infarction (see figure 8.32), the corresponding BSPM shows a negative charge at the area next to the infarction site. Referring to table 8.4, infarction No. 410 is represented by negative signals in leads V3-V6, in contrast to the transmural case (figure 8.28).

Another important conclusion from the data in table 8.4 is the existence of infarction locations which hardly change the ST-segment of standard leads. For example, infarction 522, being quite large, causes just a minor ST-depression in the V1 and V2 leads, the rest of the leads are unchanged. Infarction 621 does not cause any notable offset of the ST-segment. These infarctions are located at the postero-inferior and posterior wall close to the basis of the left ventricle, respectively. Thus the detection of these infarctions can take place only during the QRS-complex and the T-wave. Experimental measurements for patients 1 and 2 deliver quite similar results (see sections 9.3 and 9.4). For these patients no ST-segment offset has been observed.

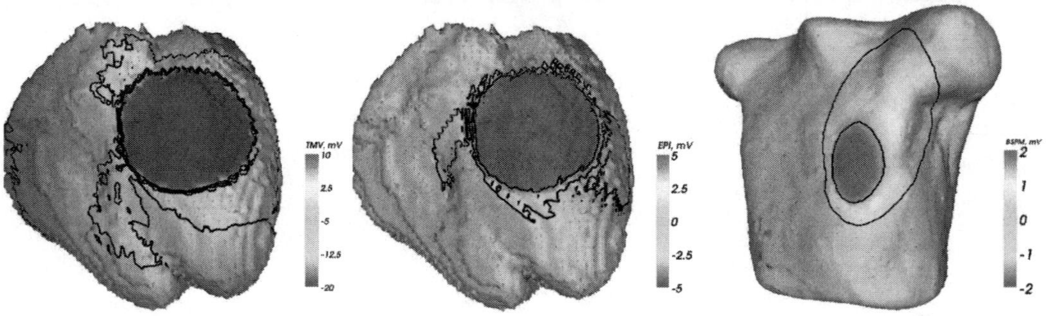

Figure 8.26: *Simulated distributions of transmembrane voltage (left), epicardial potential (center) and body surface potential (right) in the middle of the ST-segment for a patient suffering from transmural anterior infarction (index 421).*

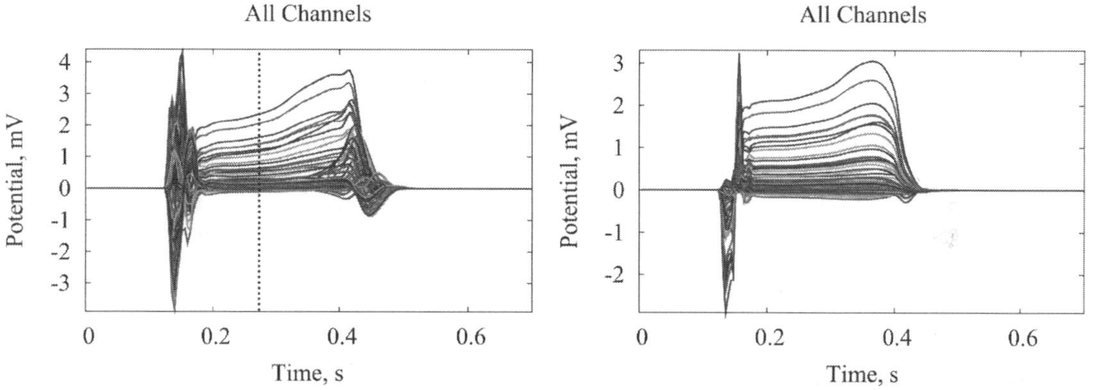

Figure 8.27: *Simulated 64-channel ECG for a patient with transmural anterior infarction (left); change of ECG caused by infarction (right). The dotted line in the simulated ECG marks the time instant at which the distributions in figure 8.26 are shown.*

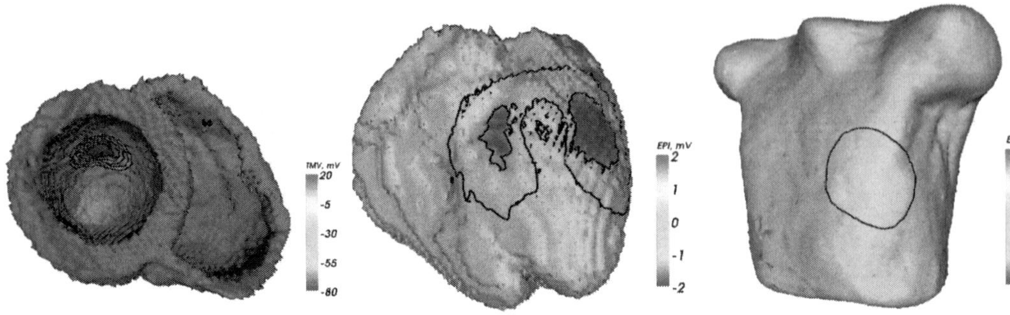

Figure 8.28: *Simulated distributions of transmembrane voltage (left), epicardial potential (center) and body surface potential (right) in the middle of the ST-segment for a patient suffering from endocardial anterior infarction (index 410).*

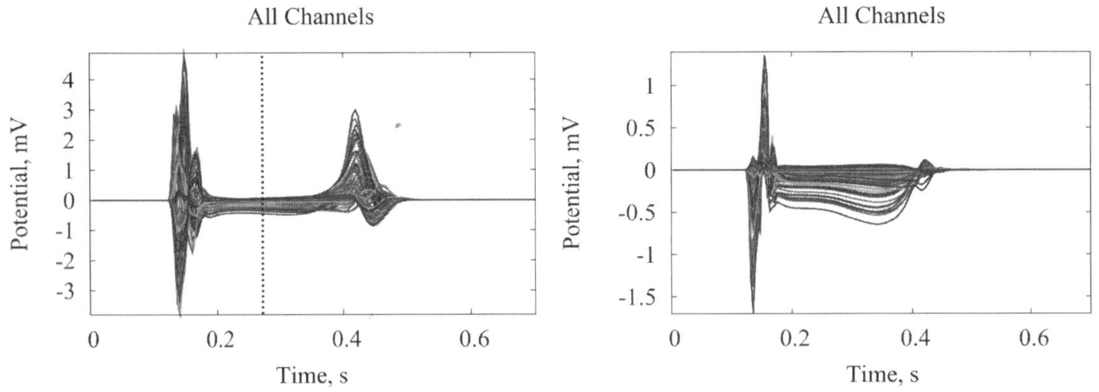

Figure 8.29: *Simulated 64-channel ECG for a patient with endocardial anterior infarction (left); change of ECG caused by this infarction (right). The dotted line marks the time instant at which the distributions in figure 8.28 are shown.*

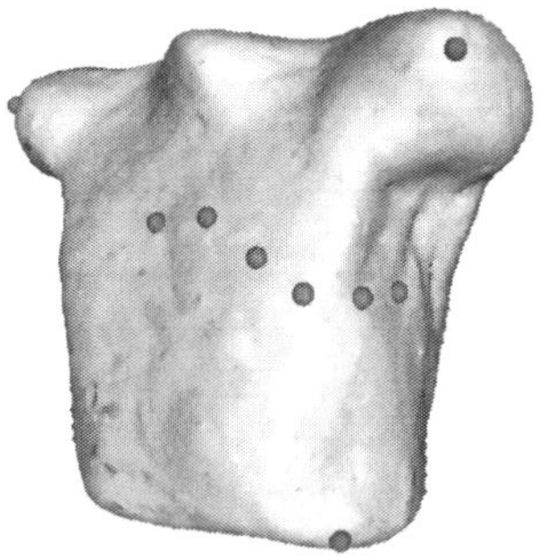

Figure 8.30: *Electrode locations selected for the measurement of standard leads.*

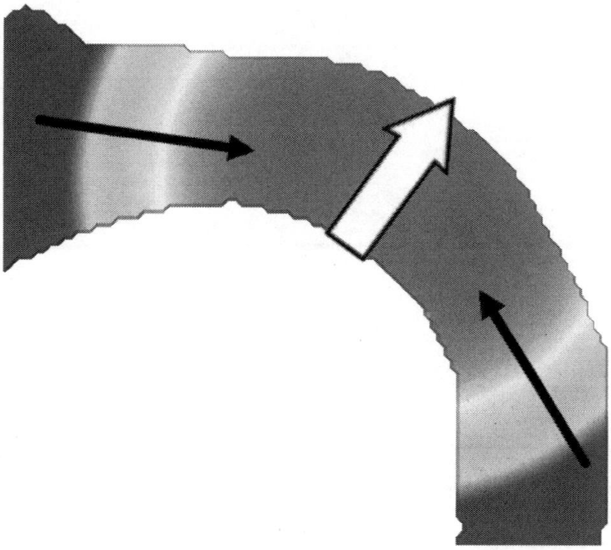

Figure 8.31: *Dipole orientation for the case of a transmural infarction. Blue color represents the negatively charged healthy myocardium, infarcted area has a positive potential (red). Black arrows represent the orientation of local dipoles towards the infarcted area. Thick white arrow shows the global dipole orientation towards the body surface.*

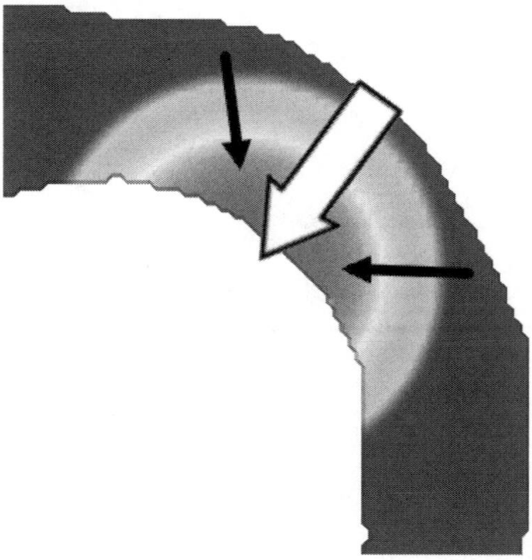

Figure 8.32: *Dipole orientation for the case of an endocardial infarction. Blue color represents the negatively charged healthy myocardium, infarcted area has a positive potential (red). Black arrows represent the orientation of local dipoles towards the infarcted area. Thick white arrow shows the global dipole orientation backwards from the body surface.*

Chapter 9

Reconstruction Results

9.1 Introduction

One test subject and 7 patients listed in section 6.1 were involved to test different methods of inverse problem solution. For each subject a finite element mesh representing the thorax anatomy was created. These meshes contain typically about 100,000 nodes and 600,000 tetrahedra. The average distance between nodes varies between 2 mm within the ventricular myocardium and up to 20 mm in large homogeneous organs. This leads to the optimal balance between memory consumption and resolution of the model.

The averaging of multiple ECG cycles in each channel was performed in order to suppress uncorrelated measurement noise. For several patients one channel delivered attenuated and strongly distorted signals, in that cases the channel was ignored.

Each data set contains the fiber orientation within the ventricular myocardium. The importance of this information is disputed (see, e.g., [167] for activation time imaging). Still the results shown in sections 7.4 (especially figure 7.7) and 8.1 prove that for the same distribution of TMV different BSPMs can be obtained depending on the anisotropy of cardiac muscle.

The inverse problem of electrocardiography is solved at least 5 times for each subject. Epicardial potentials are reconstructed using GMRes as well as Tikhonov-Greensite 0-order (TG0) regularization methods. The distributions of transmembrane voltages are reconstructed using GMRes, TG0 and Tikhonov-Greensite 2-order (TG2) regularization methods.

As these distributions have not been measured directly, the correlation between the distributions of cardiac sources reconstructed with different methods is calculated for each patient. It is assumed that a better correlation means a higher quality of the solution.

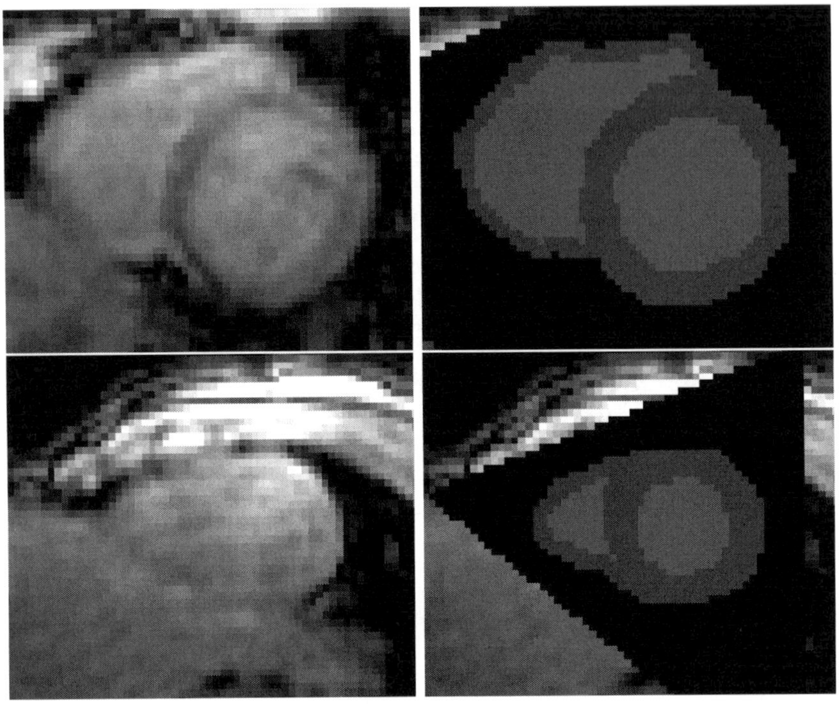

Figure 9.1: Test subject. Results of segmentation of the subject's heart (right) compared with the original SAX MRI data set (left). Top: near the ventricular base; bottom: near the apex.

9.2 Test Subject

9.2.1 Description of Subject and Segmentation Results

Test subject, M.H., male, age 20, healthy. The MRI scan of his heart in diastolic state has the resolution of $2.27 \times 2.27 \times 4\ mm^3$, that of his thorax – $5 \times 5 \times 5\ mm^3$. The anatomical model of his heart is compared with the original MRI data in figure 9.1. The volume conductor model segmented from a thorax MRI data set is compared with this data set in figure 9.2.

The anatomical model of the heart resulting from the segmentation has the resolution of $0.5 \times 0.5 \times 0.5\ mm^3$. The volume conductor model contains 109,054 nodes and 675,098 tetrahedra, the average distance between nodes varies from 2 mm within the ventricles to 10 mm elsewhere.

9.2.2 Measurement of Body Surface Potential Maps

During the measurement of his ECG the sample rate was set to 256 Hz. The resulting ECG is shown in figure 9.3. Six dotted vertical lines represent the time points at which

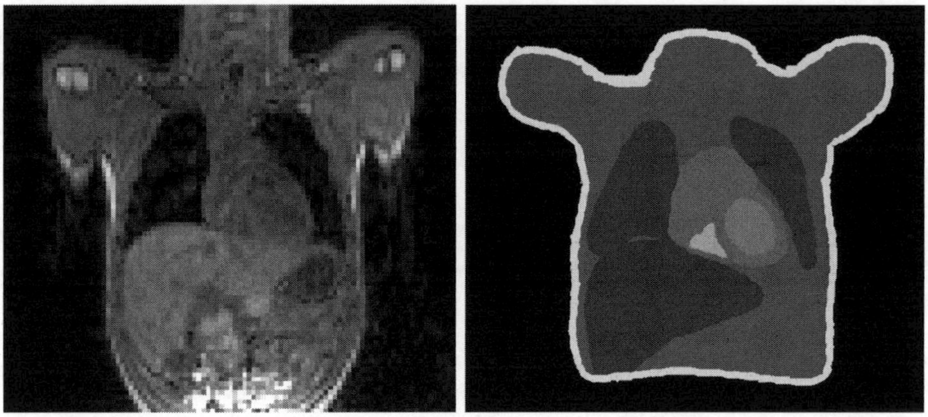

Figure 9.2: *Test subject. Anatomical model of the subject's thorax (right) compared with the original data set (left).*

the reconstructed results are shown.

The standard ECG leads are shown in figure 9.4. As there has been no electrode among the 64 channel located near to the Wilson V6 lead, this lead is not shown.

Body surface potential maps at the beginning, in the middle and at the end of the QRS-complex interpolated on the whole surface of the thorax are shown in figure 9.5. The blue color corresponds to the potential of -500 μV, the red color denotes the potential of +500 μV. Equipotential lines are shown for the potential values of -500, -300, -100, +100, +300 and +500 μV.

BSPM for the beginning, middle and end of the T-wave are shown in figure 9.10. The color scale covers the range between -0.15 and +0.15 mV, with equipotential lines displayed for -0.15, -0.05, +0.05, +0.15 mV.

9.2.3 Reconstruction of the Cardiac Sources

Two equivalent models of cardiac sources have been considered. Epicardial potentials were reconstructed using GMRes as well as Tikhonov-Greensite 0-order (TG0) regularization methods. The reconstructed distributions of epicardial potentials on the anterior surface during the QRS-complex are shown in figure 9.6. The color scale in this figure represents the range between -4 and 4 mV. Equipotential lines correspond to the potential values of -4, -2.4, -0.8, +0.8, +2.4 and +4 mV.

The same distribution from the posterolateral direction is shown in figure 9.7. As the information from this part of the heart is strongly distorted due to a larger distance to measurement electrodes, the reconstructed signals are smooth and weakened. The color range covers the EP values between -0.5 and +0.5 mV, isolines are shown for -0.5, -0.3, -0.1, +0.1, +0.3 and +0.5 mV.

Figure 9.11 demonstrates the distributions of epicardial potentials during the T-wave, anterior view. The color scale covers the range from -1 to +1 mV, with equipotential lines at -1, -0.6, -0.2, +0.2, +0.6, +1 mV.

The posterolateral view of the heart with the distribution of EP during the T-wave is shown in figure 9.12. The color range is between -0.5 and +0.5 mV, with isolines at -0.5, -0.3, ..., +0.5 mV.

The correlation between the distributions of EP reconstructed using the both regularization methods for the whole time range is shown in figure 9.15, left.

Three different regularization methods were employed to reconstruct the distributions of transmembrane voltages (TMV): GMRes, TG0 and Tikhonov-Greensite 2-order (TG2). The reconstruction results for the QRS-complex (anterior view) are shown in figure 9.8. The color scale covers the TMV range between -10 and +10 mV, equipotential lines are shown for the potential values of -10, -6, -2, +2, +6 and +10 mV.

From the posterolateral direction the distributions of TMV during the QRS-complex are shown in figure 9.9. The color scale includes values from -5 to +5 mV, with isolines at -5, -3, ..., +5 mV.

The changes of TMV during the T-wave at the anterior side of the heart are shown in figure 9.13. Here the color range covers from -3 to +3 mV, with isolines at -3, -1, +1 and +3 mV. The posterolateral side of the heart is shown in figure 9.14, color scale from -1.5 to +1.5 mV, isolines at -1.5, -0.5, +0.5, +1.5 mV.

The correlation was computed between the reconstructed TMV using TG0 vs. GMRes regularization methods (figure 9.15, center) as well as TG0 vs. TG2 methods (figure 9.15, right). The orientations of the thorax corresponding to the anterior and posterolateral views of the heart are shown in figure 9.16.

The same sets of reconstructed distributions will also be shown for all the processed patients. The diagnosis is to be derived from the comparison between the reconstructed distributions of cardiac sources for the specific patient and those for the healthy subject.

9.2.4 Conclusions

According to figure 9.15, the best and the most reliable correspondence between the solutions obtained using different regularization methods is achieved during the repolarization phase of the heart cycle. This can be easily explained: the depolarization front has a relatively small spatial spread of several mm, the corresponding spatial frequencies are quite high thus being strongly suppressed by the regularization.

During the repolarization phase, on the other hand, the distributions of transmembrane voltages are quite smooth (e.g. in figure 7.2). Thus they can be consistently reconstructed using the employed regularization methods.

Considering the repolarization of the heart in figures 9.11 and 9.13, it can be seen that the repolarization starts at the base of the right ventricle as well as on the epicardial anterior surface of the left ventricle, which is in a good correspondence with the results obtained by van Oosterom in [33].

Also the model-based approach shown in chapter 8 delivers results quite similar to those shown in this section.

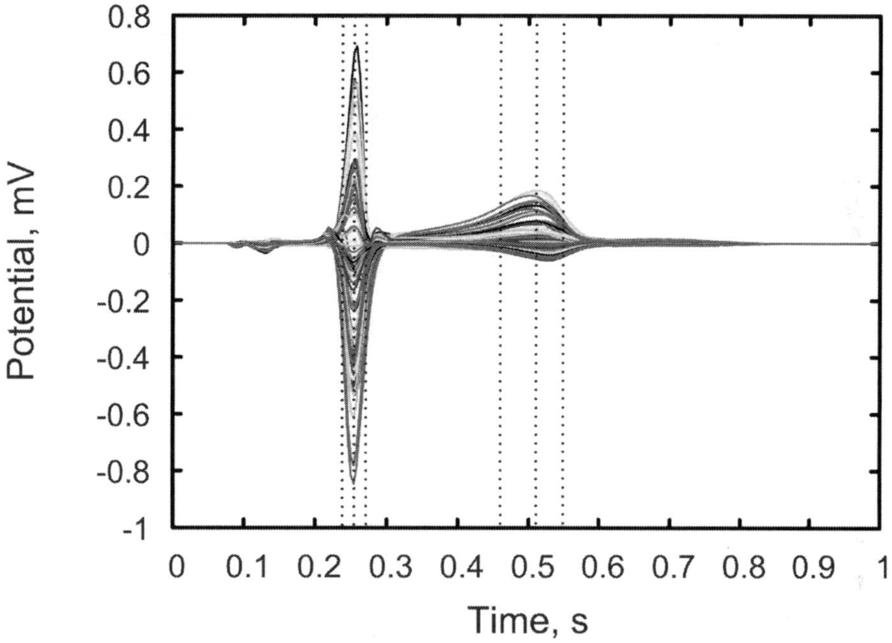

Figure 9.3: *Test subject. ECG recorded with 64 measurement electrodes. Vertical dotted lines represent the time points at which the reconstruction was performed.*

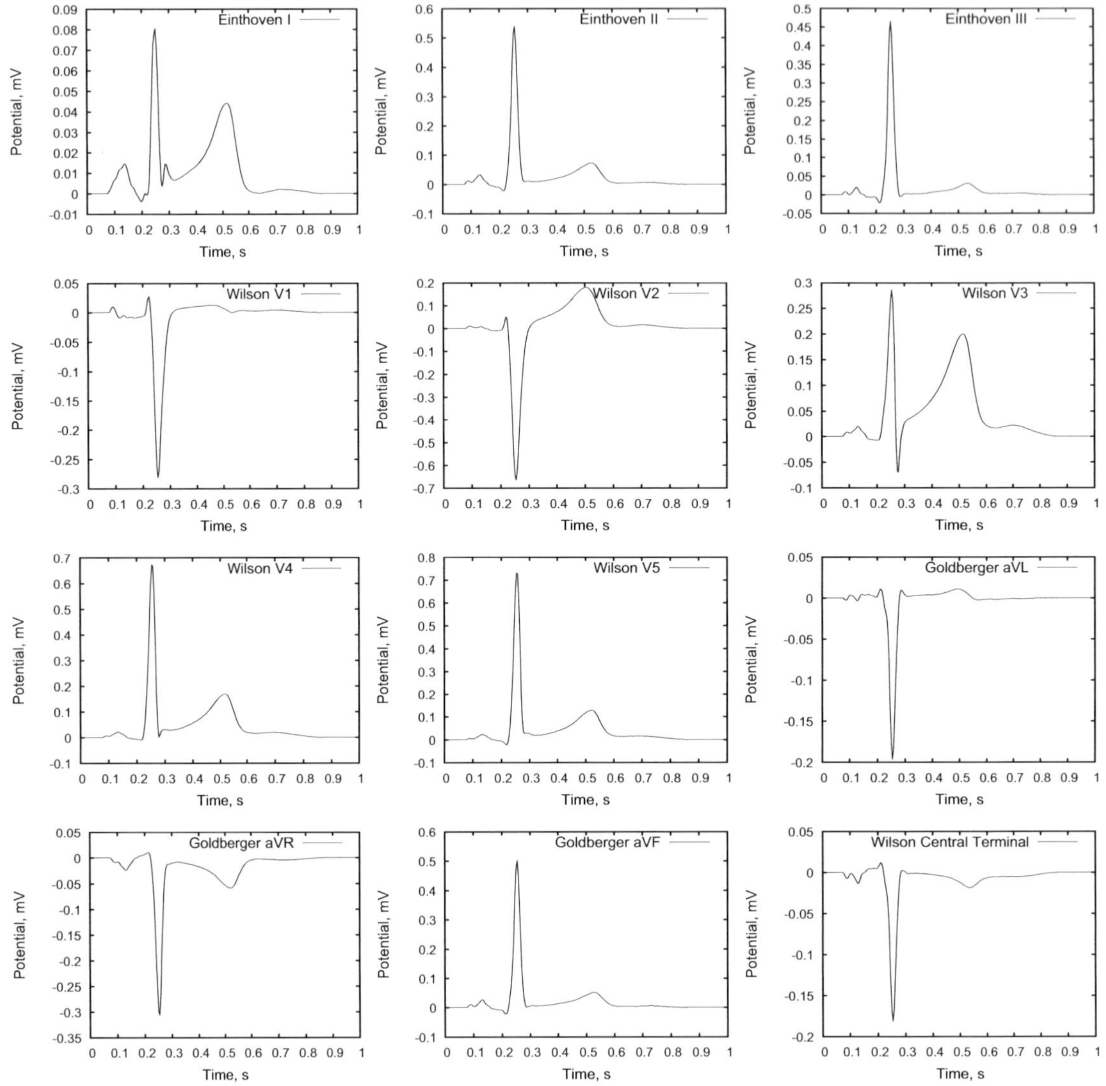

Figure 9.4: *Test subject. Einthoven, Goldberger and Wilson standard leads are shown. There was no lead among the electrodes near enough to the standard electrode location V6.*

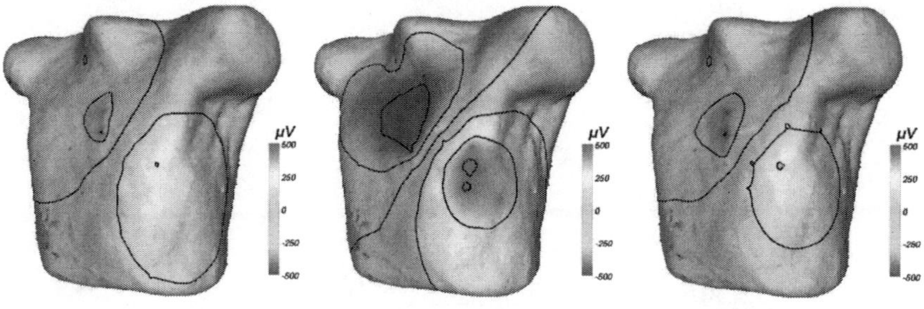

Figure 9.5: *Test subject. Body surface potential maps (BSPM) during the QRS-complex.*

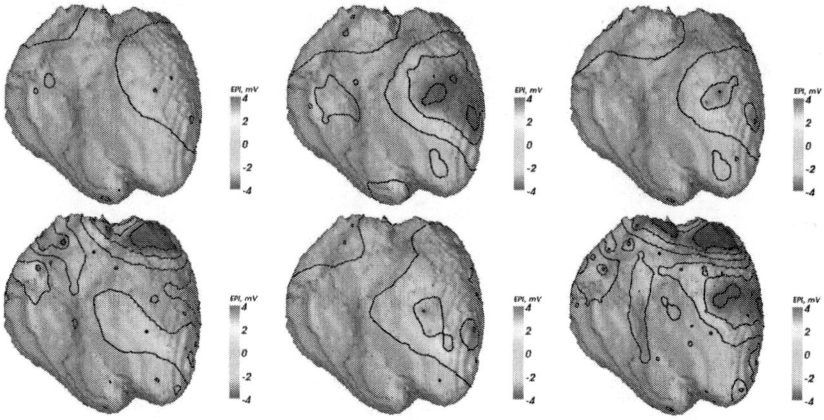

Figure 9.6: *Distributions of EP reconstructed from the measured BSPMs using GMRes (top) as well as TG0 (bottom) regularizations for the QRS-complex. Anterior view.*

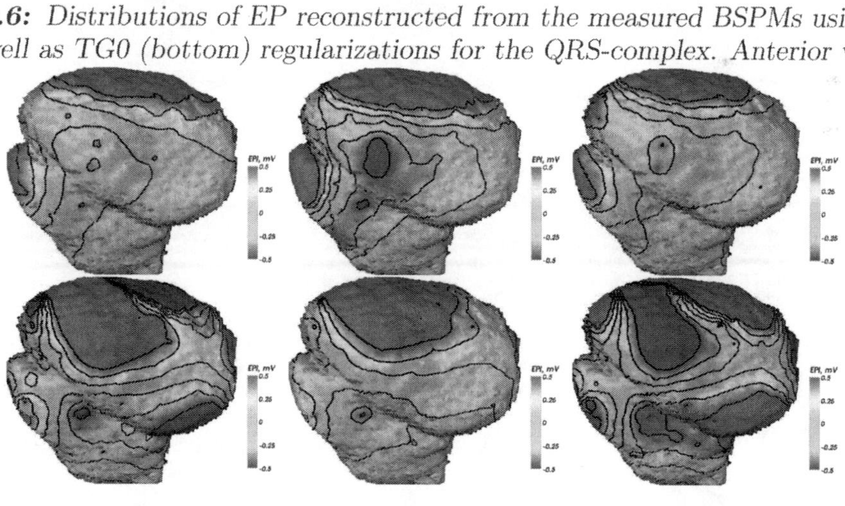

Figure 9.7: *Distributions of EP reconstructed from the measured BSPMs using GMRes (top) as well as TG0 (bottom) regularizations for the QRS-complex. Posterolateral view.*

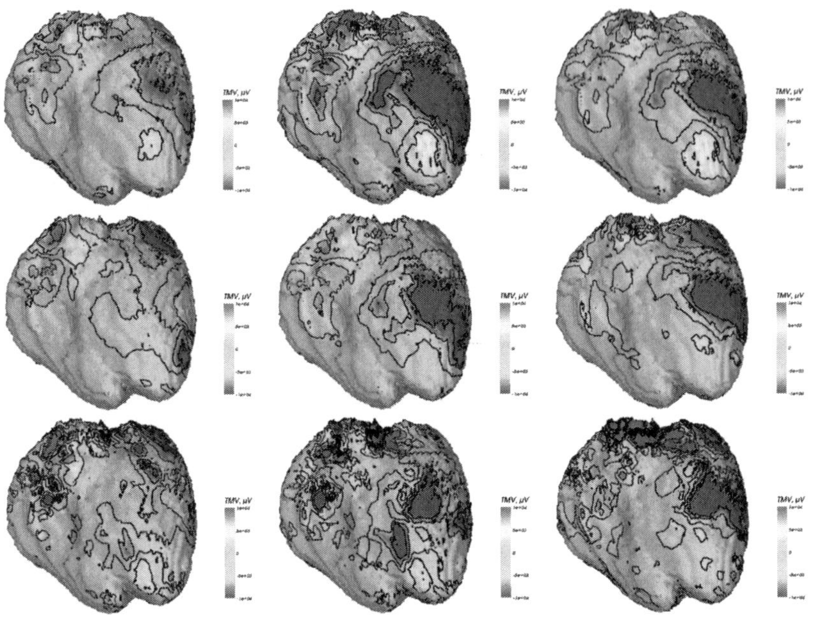

Figure 9.8: *Distributions of TMV reconstructed from the measured BSPMs using GM-Res (top), TG0 (middle) as well as TG2 (bottom) regularizations for the QRS-complex. Anterior view.*

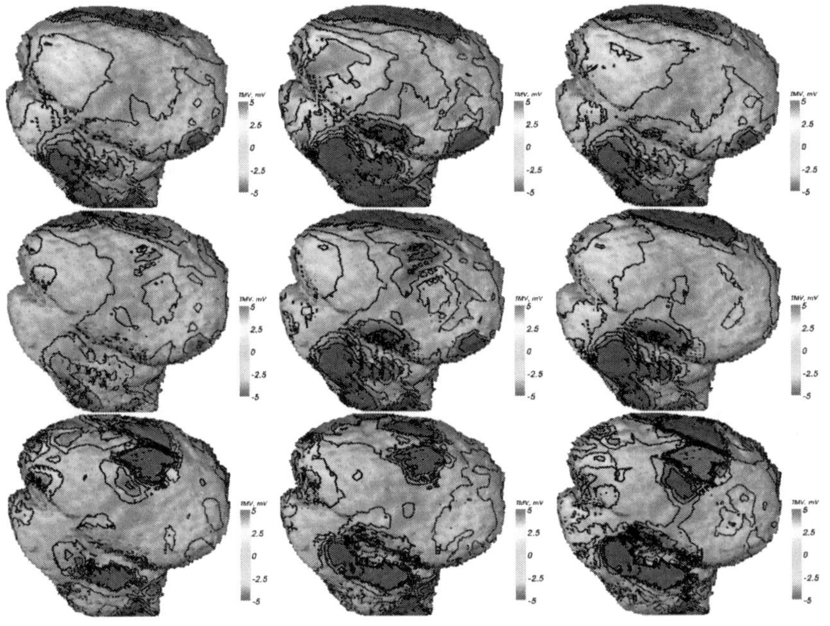

Figure 9.9: *Distributions of TMV reconstructed from the measured BSPMs using GM-Res (top), TG0 (middle) as well as TG2 (bottom) regularizations for the QRS-complex. Posterolateral view.*

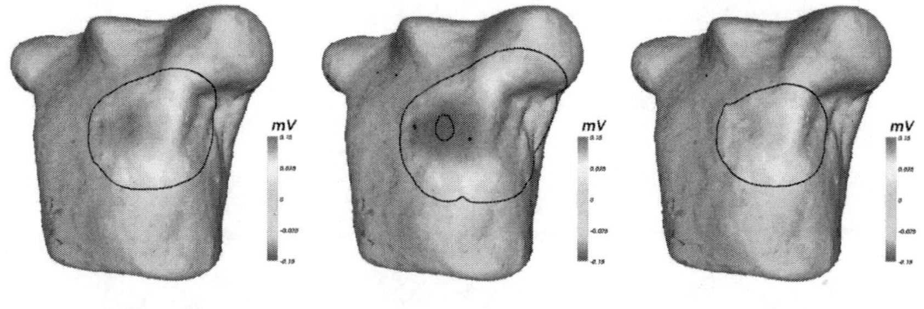

Figure 9.10: *Test subject. BSPM during the T-wave.*

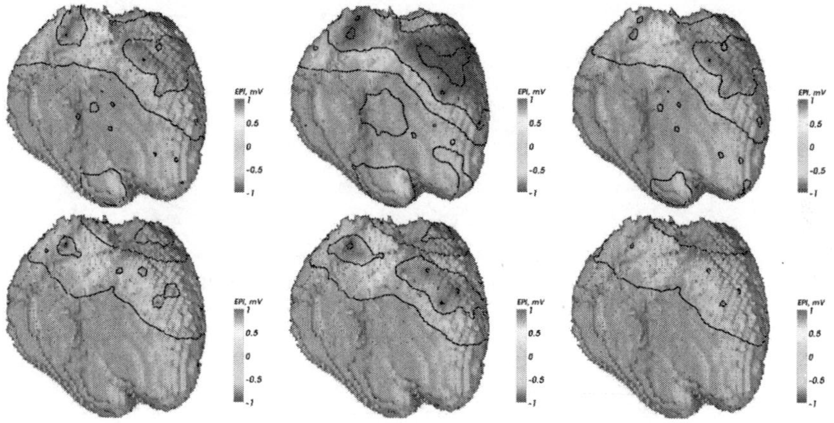

Figure 9.11: *Distributions of EP reconstructed from the measured BSPMs using GMRes regularization (top) as well as TG0 regularization (bottom) during the T-wave. Anterior view.*

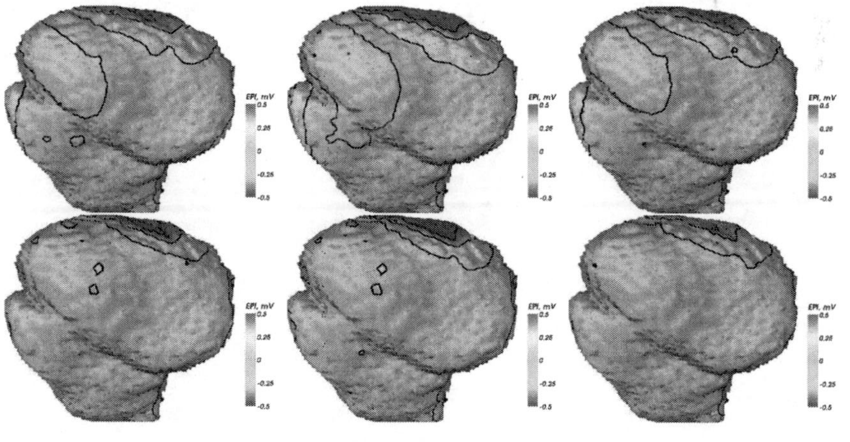

Figure 9.12: *Distributions of EP reconstructed from the measured BSPMs using GMRes regularization (top) as well as TG0 regularization (bottom) during the T-wave. Posterolateral view.*

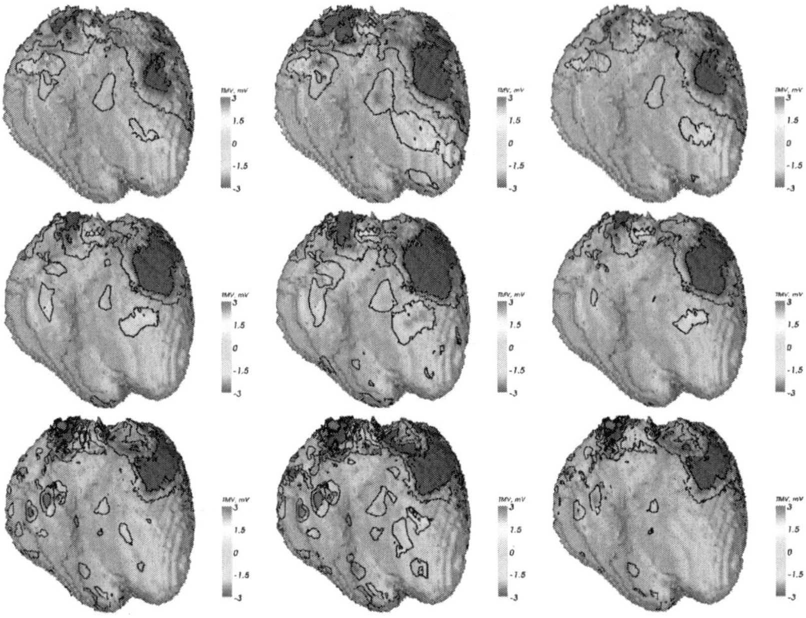

Figure 9.13: *Distributions of TMV reconstructed from the measured BSPMs using GMRes (top), TG0 (middle) as well as TG2 (bottom) regularizations during the T-wave. Anterior view.*

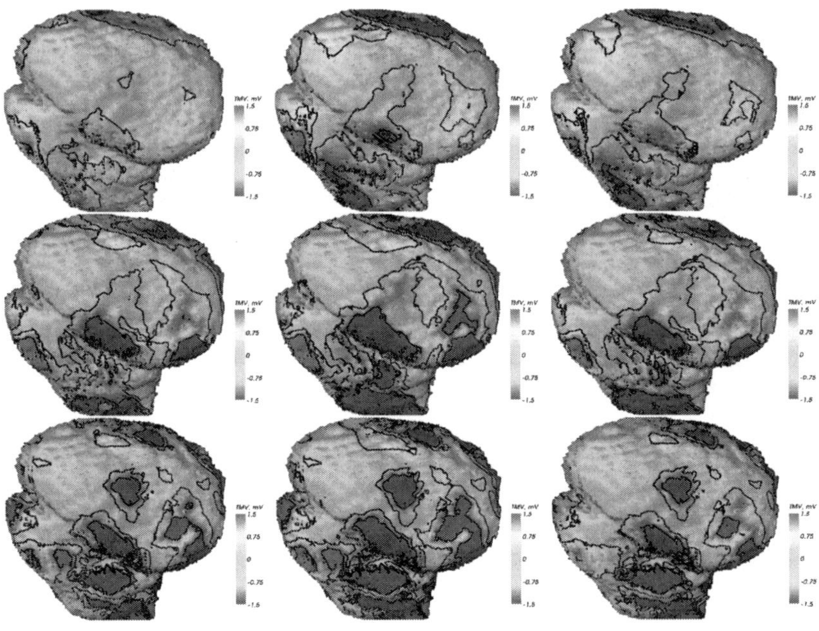

Figure 9.14: *Distributions of TMV reconstructed from the measured BSPMs using GMRes (top), TG0 (middle) as well as TG2 (bottom) regularizations during the T-wave. Posterolateral view.*

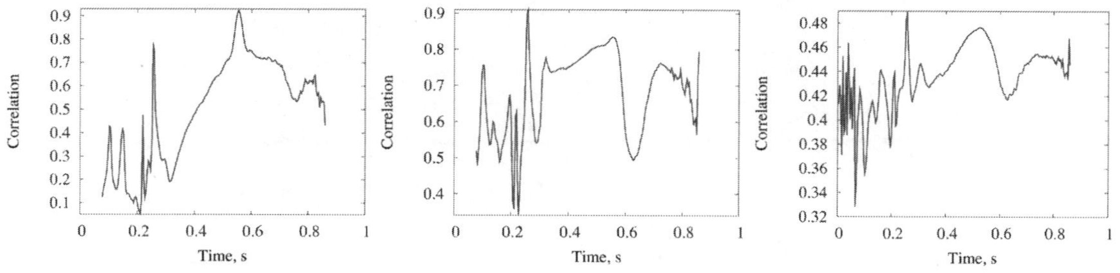

Figure 9.15: *Test subject. Correlation between the reconstructed EP using GMRes vs. TG0 regularizations (left); between TMV distributions using GMRes vs. TG0 regularizations (center); using TG2 vs. TG0 regularizations (right).*

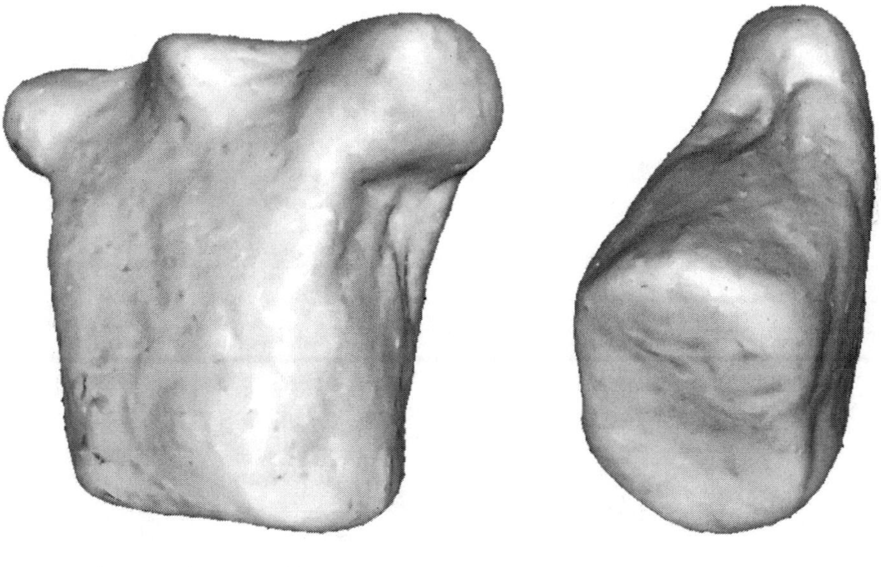

Figure 9.16: *Test subject. Thorax orientation corresponding to that of the heart: anterior view (left), posterior view (right).*

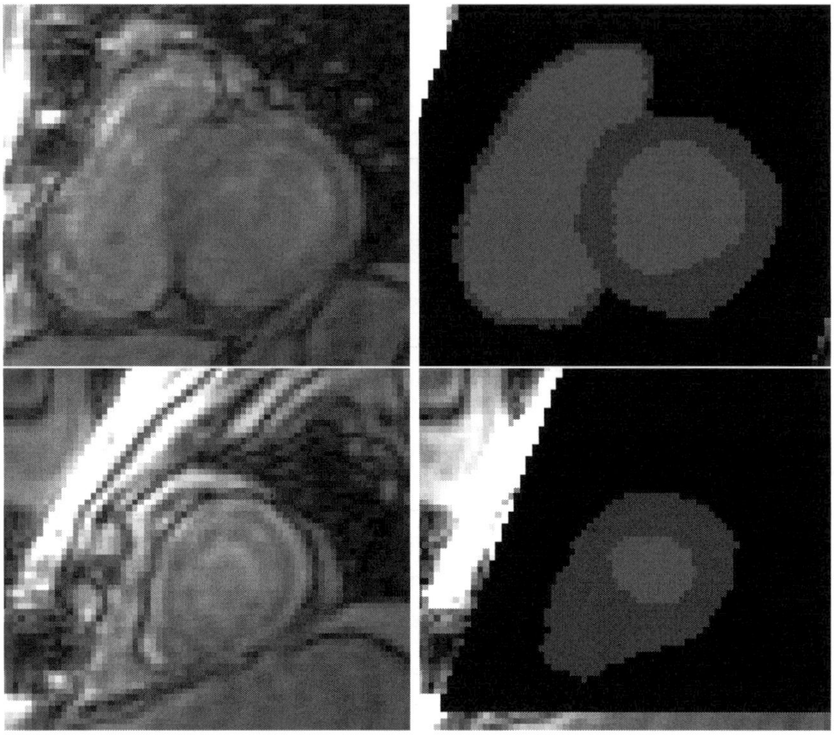

Figure 9.17: *Patient 1. Results of segmentation of the subject's heart (right) compared with the original SAX MRI data set (left). Top: near the ventricular base; bottom: near the apex.*

9.3 Patient 1

9.3.1 Description of the Patient and Segmentation Results

Patient 1, E.L., male, age 63, an old posterior infarction is diagnosed. Resolution of the heart MRI data set was $2.27 \times 2.27 \times 4\ mm^3$, thorax – $4 \times 4 \times 4\ mm^3$. The anatomical model of the patient's heart is compared with the original MRI data in figure 9.17, the segmentation of the thorax is shown in figure 9.18.

The anatomical model of the heart was created with the resolution of $1 \times 1 \times 1\ mm^3$ and contained 249,434 excitable voxels. The atria were not segmented due to the lacking resolution of MRI data.

The finite element mesh of the thorax model contains 89,107 nodes and 544,421 tetrahedra, with 51,549 nodes belonging to the ventricular myocardium, with the average distance between nodes of 2 mm in this area. This model includes heart, lungs, liver, stomach, spleen and kidneys.

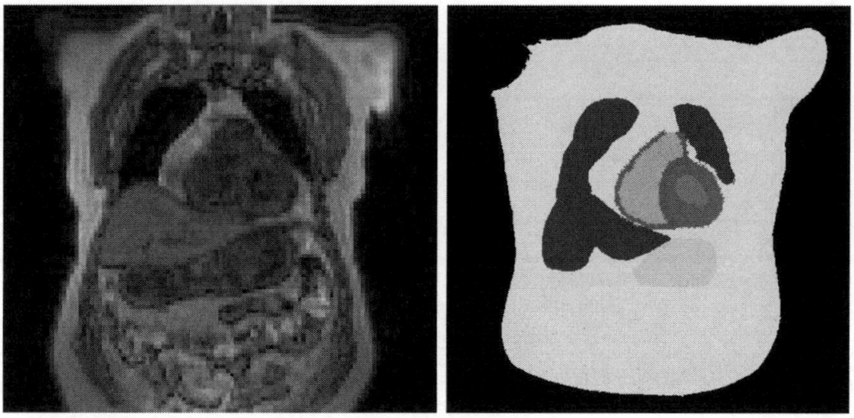

Figure 9.18: *Patient 1. Anatomical model of the subject's thorax (right) compared with the original data set (left).*

9.3.2 Measurement of BSPM

The 64-channel ECG was recorded with the BioSemi system. The sample rate was set to 2048 Hz. A plot with all the channels of ECG is shown in figure 9.19. In this figure the time points are shown, at which the inverse problem solutions are presented.

The standard leads of ECG are shown in figure 9.20. The ECG was recorded during 200 s, single ECG cycles were cut out, superimposed and averaged as described in section 6.3.

The BSPM at the beginning, in the middle and at the end of QRS complex, interpolated on the surface of the mesh, are shown in figure 9.21. Same potential distributions during the T-wave are shown in figure 9.26. The potential distributions during the T-wave are shown with a smaller color range than those during the QRS-complex, as the amplitude of the T-wave in this case was much smaller.

The comparison between the BSPMs of a healthy subject (figure 9.5) and those of this patient shows that the orientation of the cardiac dipole is higher for the patient, with a larger change during the QRS. According to [38], this is a typical sign of a posteroinferior infarction.

The distribution of body surface potentials during the T-wave do not show any clear differences. As the infarction scar is quite old, no visible offset of the ST-segment is detected.

9.3.3 Reconstruction Results

The correlation between the solutions of inverse problem employing different regularization methods for this patient (figure 9.31) is quite high both during the QRS-complex and the T-wave, thus an assumption could be made that the solution is correct for the both time intervals.

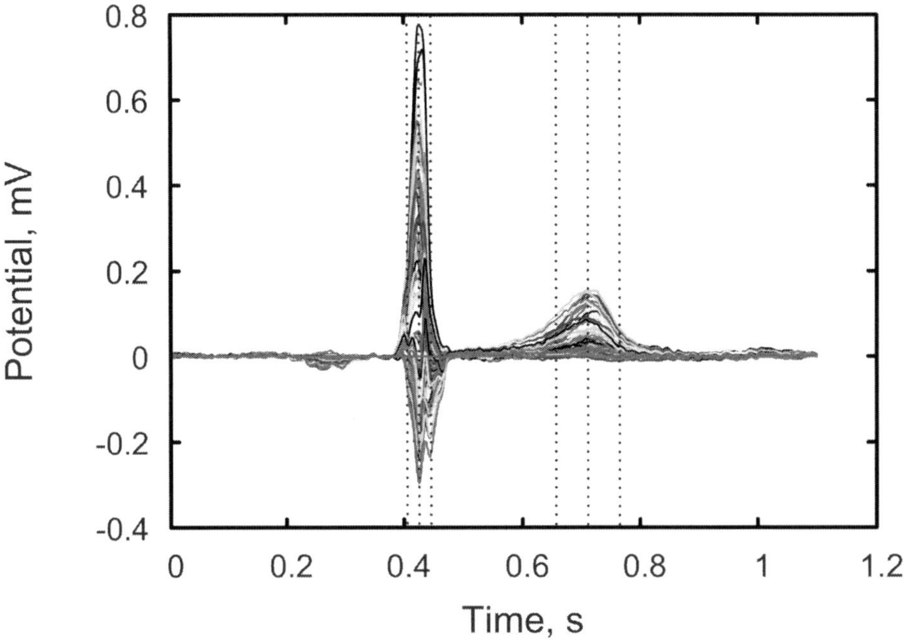

Figure 9.19: *Patient 1. ECG recorded with 64 measurement electrodes. Vertical dotted lines represent the time points at which the reconstruction was performed.*

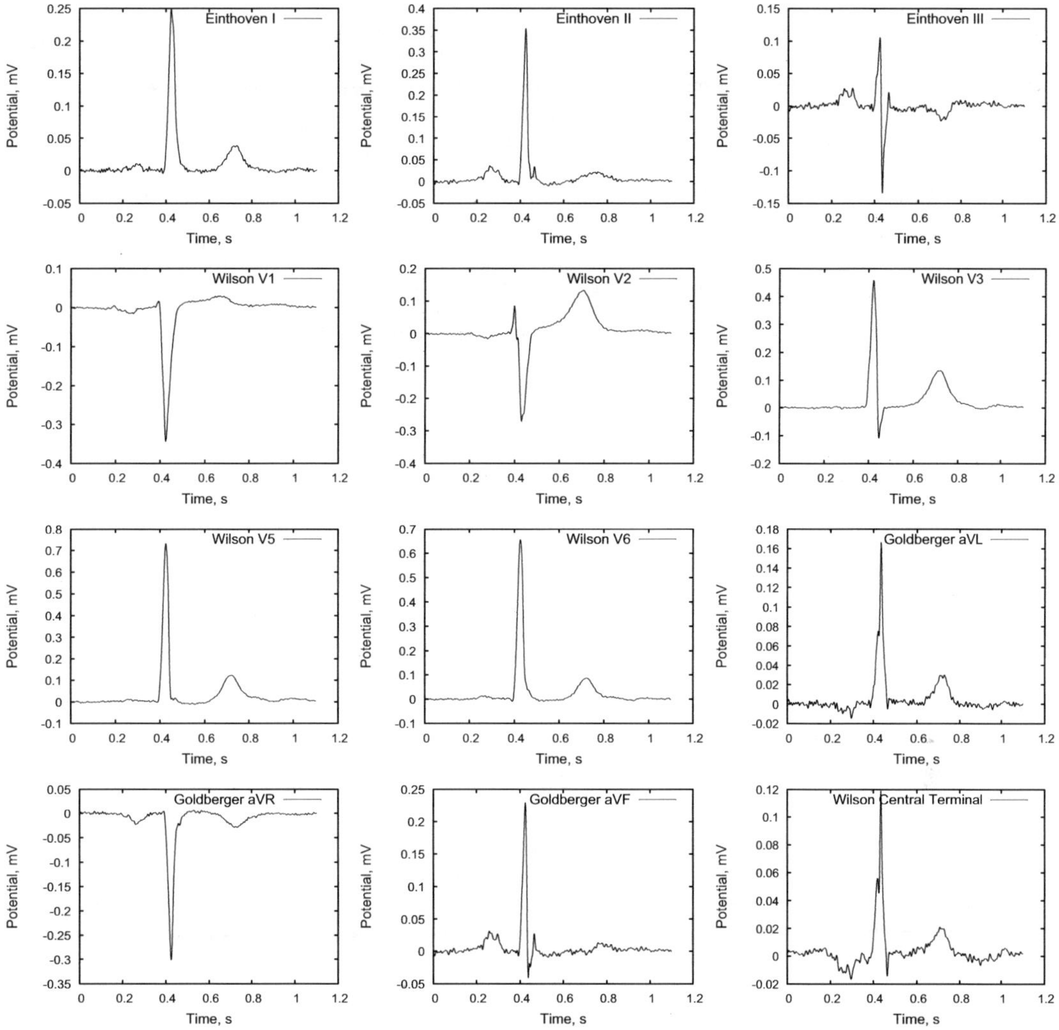

Figure 9.20: *Patient 1. Locations of the standard leads; 64-channel ECG; standard leads, measured on the test subject 2. There was no lead among the electrodes near enough to the standard electrode location V4.*

Figures 9.22 and 9.23 show the reconstructed distributions of epicardial potentials during the QRS-complex – anterior and posterior views, correspondingly. Different color scales were chosen for these views, from -3 to +3 mV for the anterior and from -1.5 to +1.5 mV for the posterior view. The reason consists in the absence of measurement electrodes on the back of the patient. Thus the sources in the posterior part of the heart are strongly smoothed by the regularization.

In figures 9.24 and 9.25 the reconstructed distributions of TMV are depicted also on the anterior and posterior sides of the heart. In this case it was possible to use the same color scale in the both cases – from -5 to +5 mV.

The distributions of epicardial potentials during the T-wave are shown in figures 9.27 and 9.28 (again, anterior and posterior views, correspondingly.) The color scale was chosen between -1 and +1 mV for the anterior and between -0.5 and +0.5 mV for the posterior view.

Finally, the distributions of TMV during the T-wave for the both views are shown in figures 9.29 and 9.30. In the both cases the color scale was chosen between -1 and +1 mV.

Figure 9.32 shows the thorax observed from the directions corresponding to the anterior and posterior views of the heart. This figure is provided for better understanding of the heart orientation.

9.3.4 Conclusions

A large positive area at the lateral side of the left ventricle can be seen, quite similar to that in the case of the healthy subject (see figure 9.6). Still a small area with positive epicardial potentials can be distinguished in the posterior view, which might correspond to the infarction scar.

Considering the reconstructed distributions of transmembrane voltages for the same time interval in figures 9.24 and 9.25, the same area appears to possess a smaller TMV than the regions around it.

The same region remains suspicious during the T-wave. Figures 9.28 and 9.30 show an area with a lower TMV (and, correspondingly, with a higher EP). Thus an infarction in this region can be assumed.

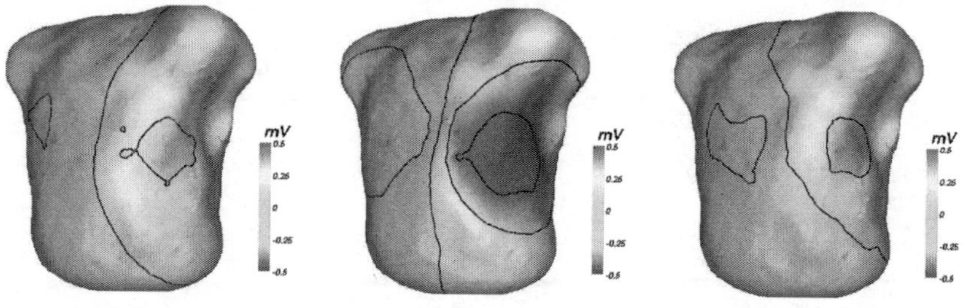

Figure 9.21: *Patient 1. Body surface potential maps (BSPM) during the QRS-complex.*

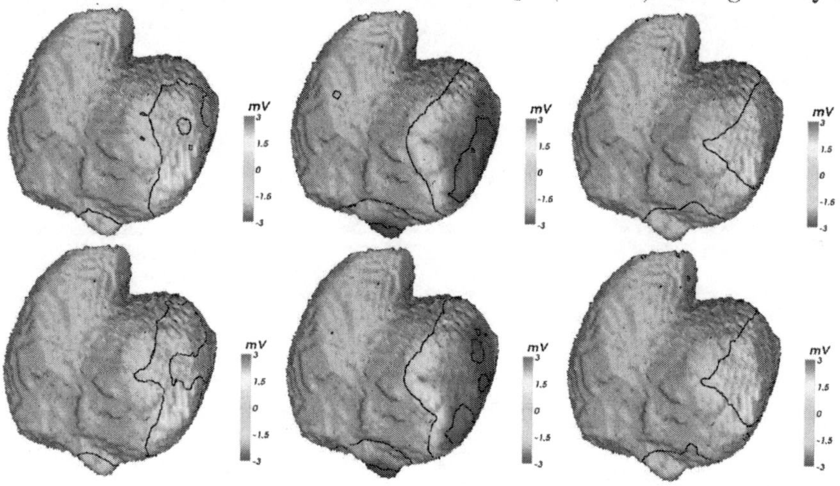

Figure 9.22: *Distributions of EP reconstructed from the measured BSPMs using GMRes (top) as well as TG0 (bottom) regularizations. Anterior view.*

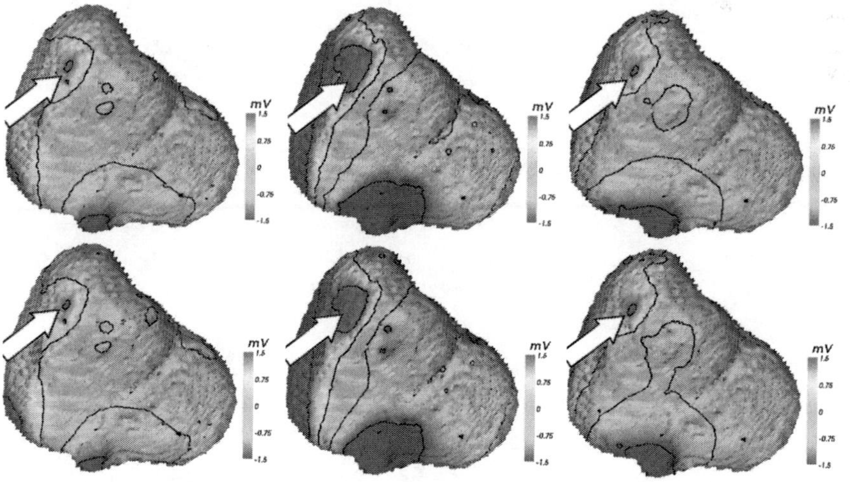

Figure 9.23: *Distributions of EP reconstructed from the measured BSPMs using GMRes (top) as well as TG0 (bottom) regularizations. Posterior view.*

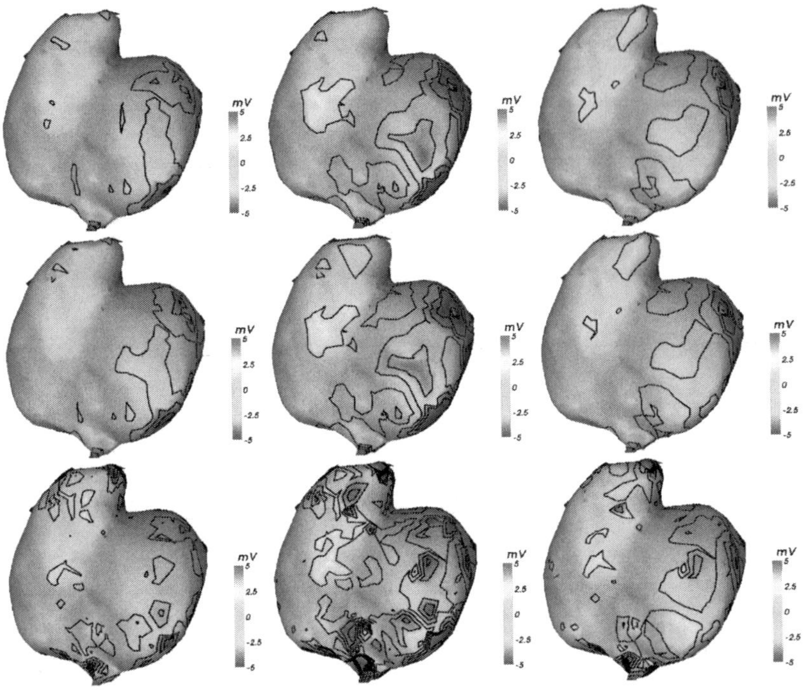

Figure 9.24: *Distributions of TMV reconstructed from the measured BSPMs using GM-Res (top), TG0 (middle) as well as TG2 (bottom) regularizations. Anterior view.*

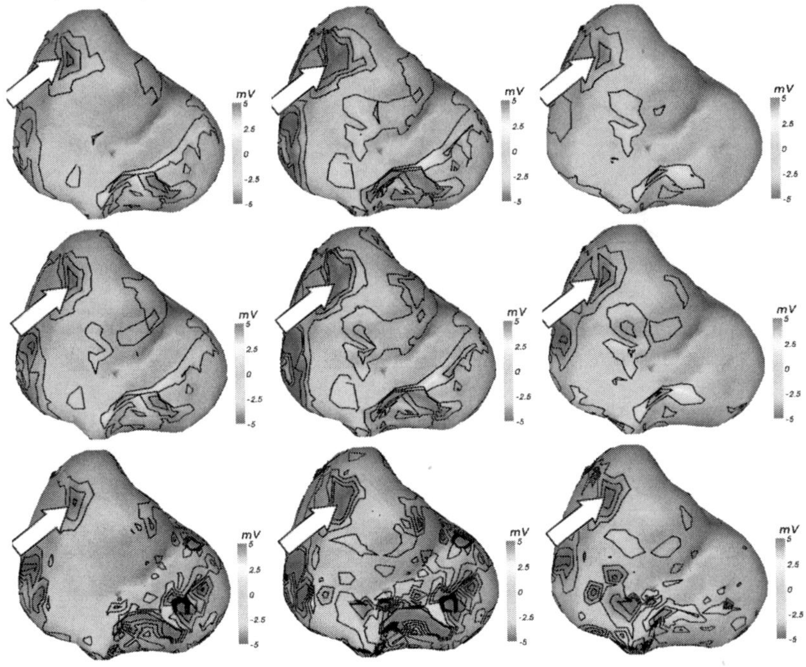

Figure 9.25: *Distributions of TMV reconstructed from the measured BSPMs using GM-Res (top), TG0 (middle) as well as TG2 (bottom) regularizations. Posterior view.*

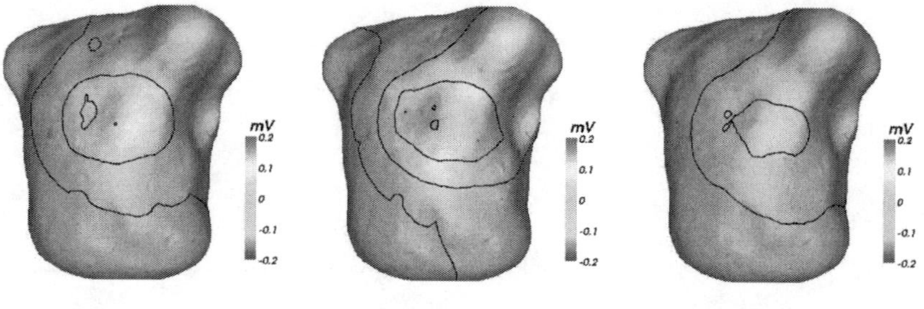

Figure 9.26: *Patient 1. BSPM during the T-wave.*

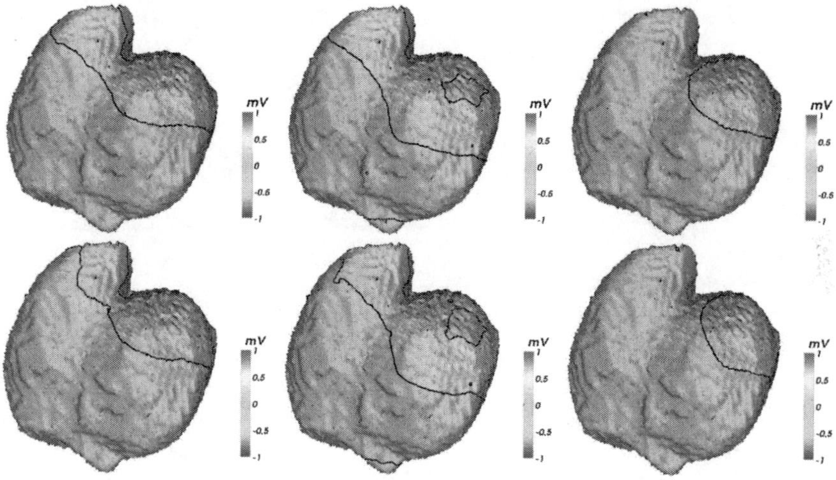

Figure 9.27: *Distributions of EP reconstructed from the measured BSPMs using GMRes regularization (top) as well as TG0 regularization (bottom). Anterior view.*

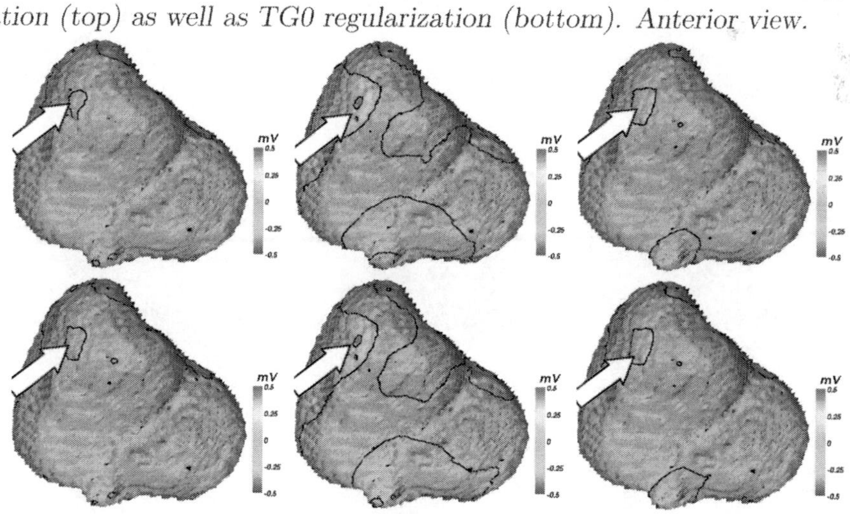

Figure 9.28: *Distributions of EP reconstructed from the measured BSPMs using GMRes regularization (top) as well as TG0 regularization (bottom). Posterior view.*

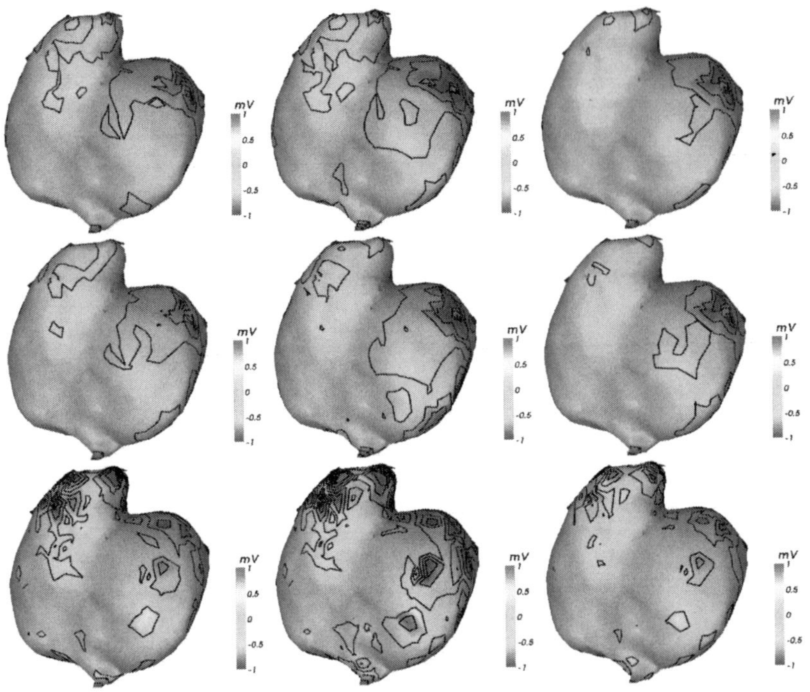

Figure 9.29: *Distributions of TMV reconstructed from the measured BSPMs using GM-Res (top), TG0 (middle) as well as TG2 (bottom) regularizations. Anterior view.*

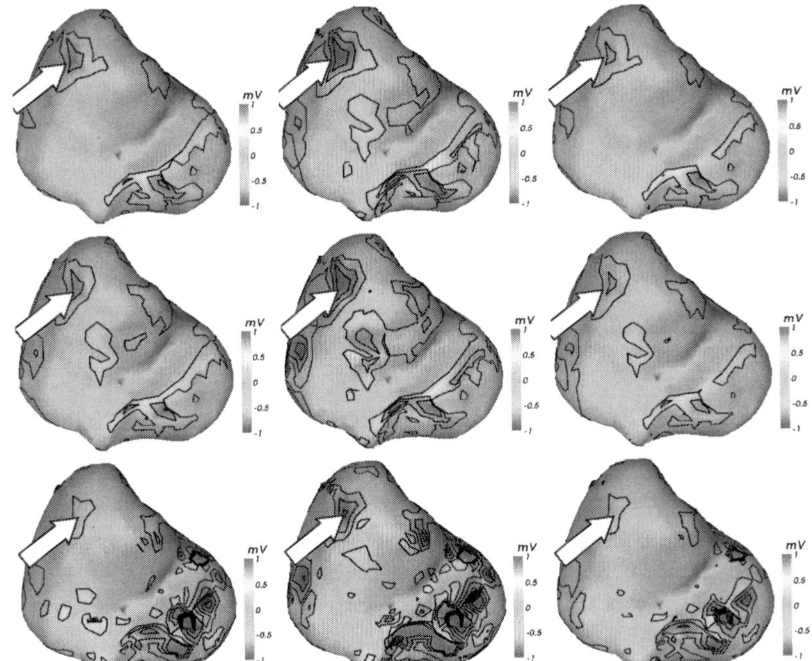

Figure 9.30: *Distributions of TMV reconstructed from the measured BSPMs using GM-Res (top), TG0 (middle) as well as TG2 (bottom) regularizations. Posterior view.*

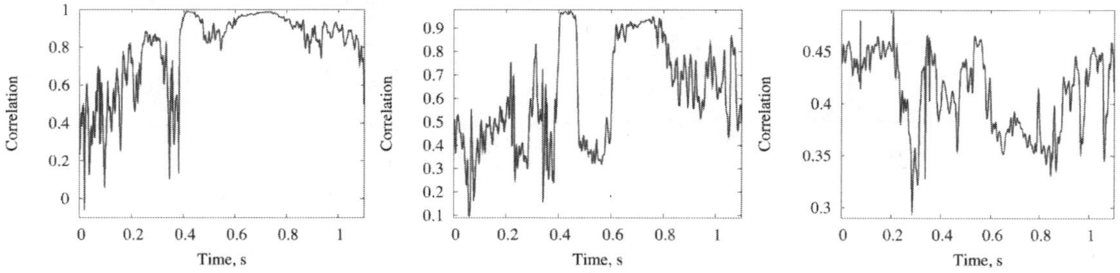

Figure 9.31: *Patient 1. Correlation between the reconstructed EP using GMRes vs. TG0 regularizations (left); between TMV distributions using GMRes vs. TG0 regularizations (middle); using TG2 vs. TG0 regularizations (right).*

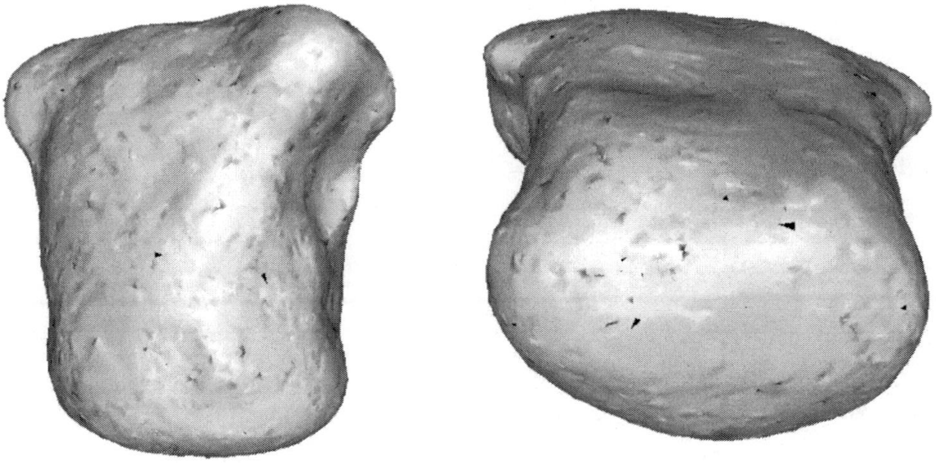

Figure 9.32: *Patient 1. Thorax orientation corresponding to that of the heart: anterior view (left), posterior view (right).*

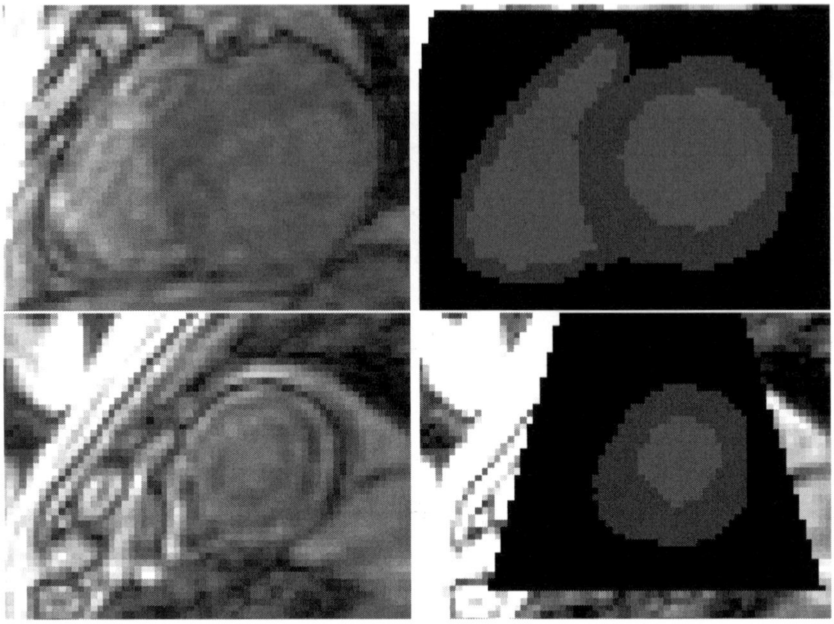

Figure 9.33: *Patient 2. Results of segmentation of the subject's heart (right) compared with the original SAX MRI data set (left). Top: near the ventricular base; bottom: near the apex.*

9.4 Patient 2

9.4.1 Description of the Patient and Segmentation Results

Patient 2, P.K., male, age 61, posterior and posterolateral infarctions are diagnosed. Resolution of the heart MRI data set was $2.27 \times 2.27 \times 4\ mm^3$, thorax – $4 \times 4 \times 4\ mm^3$.

The anatomical model of the heart has the resolution of $1 \times 1 \times 1\ mm^3$ and contains 279374 excitable voxels. This model does not include atria. In figure 9.33 the model is compared with the original MRI data.

The finite element model of the patient's thorax contains 84,611 nodes and 516,712 tetrahedra. The resolution of the mesh reproducing myocardial tissue is 2 mm. Lungs, heart, liver, spleen, stomach and kidneys are included. A cross section of the segmented thorax as well as the corresponding MR image are shown in figure 9.34.

9.4.2 Measurement of BSPM

The 64-channel ECG was recorded with the BioSemi system. The sample rate was set to 2048 Hz. A plot with all the channels of ECG as well as the standard leads of ECG are shown in figure 9.35. The ECG was recorded during 200 s. The same averaging procedure was performed to filter out the measurement noise.

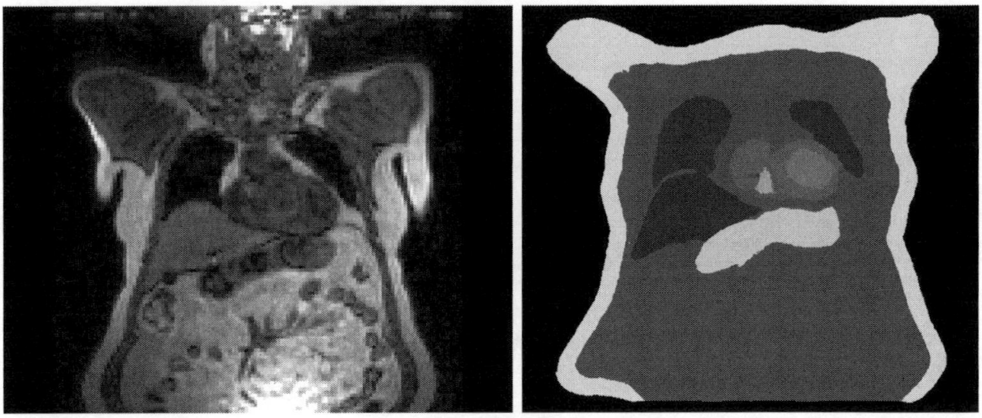

Figure 9.34: *Patient 2. Anatomical model of the subject's thorax (right) compared with the original data set (left).*

It can be clearly seen in figure 9.35, that one electrode has delivered a strongly attenuated signal distorted with a large noise. This might be caused by a poor electrical contact between the electrode and body surface or by some hardware problem. This channel was not used for reconstruction of cardiac sources.

Six vertical dotted lines in this figure indicate the time points at which the BSPMs as well as the corresponding solutions of inverse problem of electrocardiography are shown.

From the set of 64 electrodes those located near the standard locations were selected, standard leads (Wilson, Goldberger and Einthoven) are shown in figure 9.36.

Figure 9.37 shows measured BSPMs at the beginning, in the middle and at the end of the QRS-complex. Body surface potential distributions during the T-wave are shown in figure 9.37.

9.4.3 Reconstruction Results

The correlation between the results provided by different regularization methods (figure 9.47) has its maxima during the QRS-complex and T-wave, reaching 0.7 for epicardial potentials and up to 0.9 during the T-wave for TMV distributions. If the measured signal is small, the correlation is small as well, because the reconstructed distribution is primarily defined by the measurement noise.

Figures 9.38 and 9.39 represent the reconstructed distributions of epicardial potentials during the T-wave observed from anterior and posteriorlateral directions, respectively. The color scale includes the range between -1.5 and +1.5 mV for the anterior view and from -0.75 to +0.75 mV for the posterolateral view.

The reconstructed distributions of TMV during the QRS-complex are shown in figures 9.40 and 9.41 – anterior and posterolateral views, respectively. The color scale includes the range between -3 and +3 mV.

The distributions of epicardial potentials during the T-wave are shown in figures 9.43

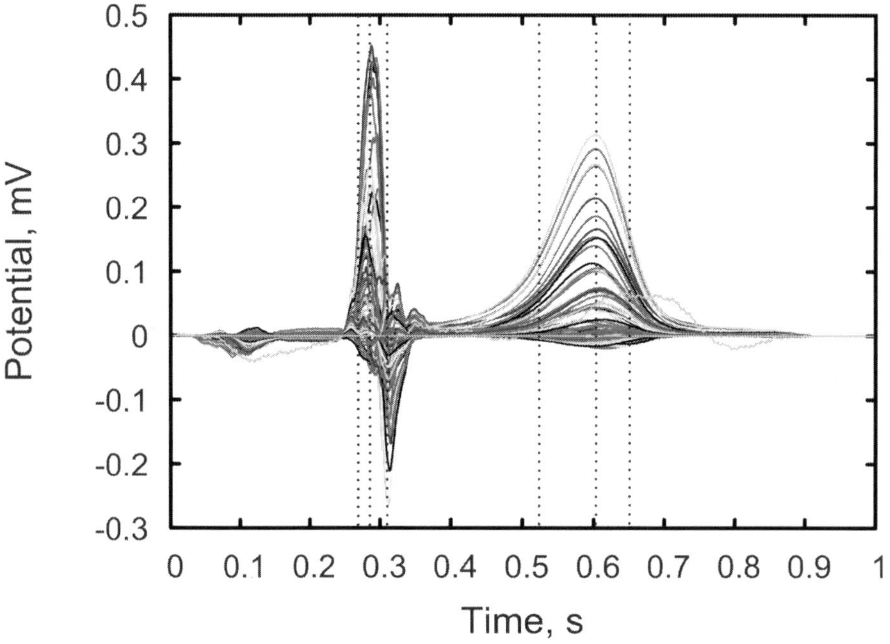

Figure 9.35: *Patient 2. ECG recorded with 64 measurement electrodes. One channel (shown with a green line) obviously delivers a distorted signal. Vertical dotted lines represent the time points at which the reconstruction was performed.*

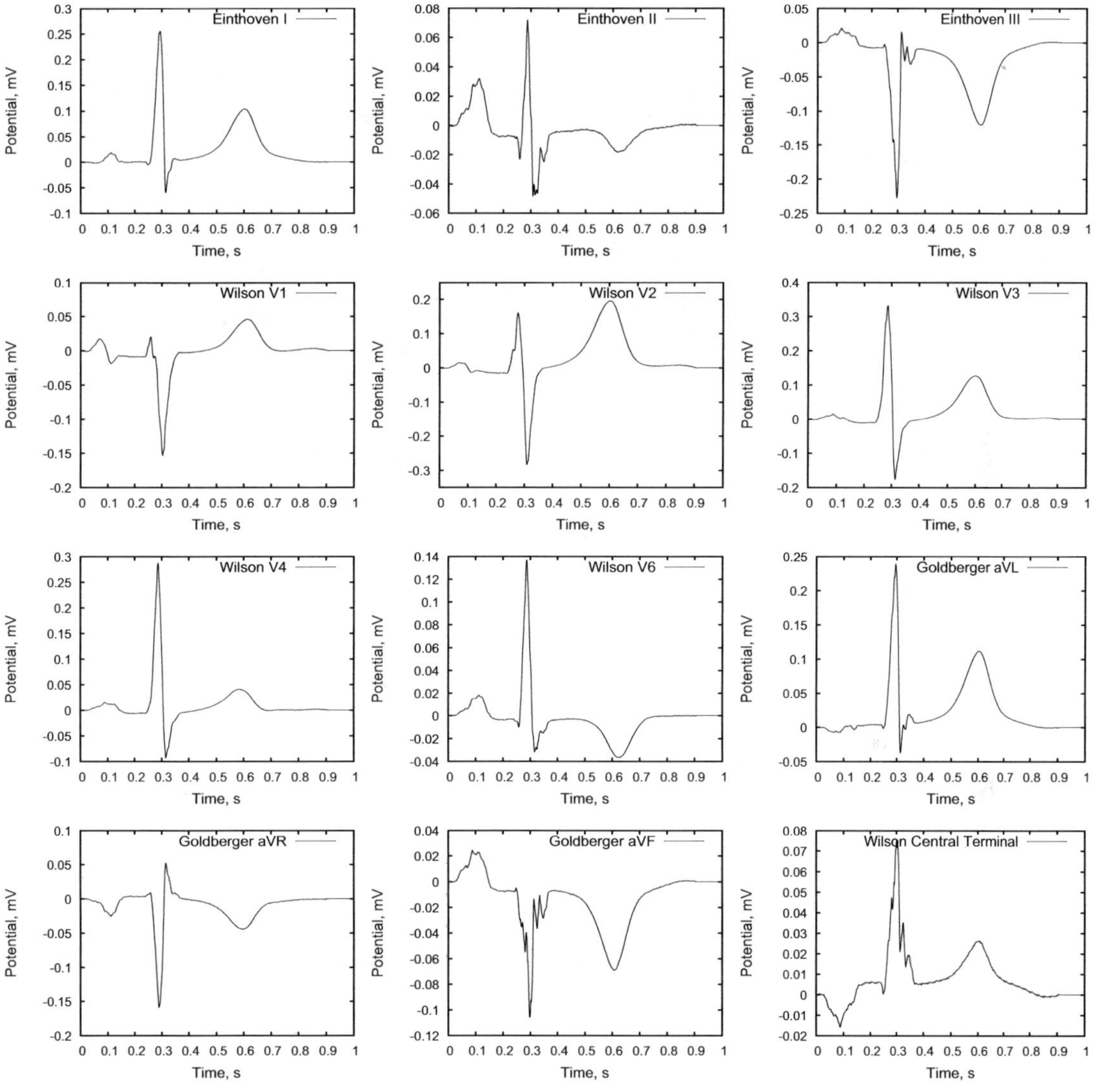

Figure 9.36: *Patient 2. Locations of the standard leads; 64-channel ECG; standard leads. There was no lead among the electrodes near enough to the standard electrode location V5.*

and 9.44. In this case the color scale covers the range between -1.5 and +1.5 mV for the anterior view (figure 9.43), whereas the in the posterior view the range is from -0.75 to +0.75 mV.

In figures 9.45 and 9.46 the distributions of TMV during the T-wave are shown. In both figures the color scale is chosen to include the range between -3 and +3 mV.

Figure 9.48 demonstrates the thorax of the patient observed from the same direction as the heart in anterior and posterolateral views.

9.4.4 Conclusions

As the correlation in figure 9.47 is quite high (almost 1.0 for TMV reconstruction using GMRes vs. TG0) during the T-wave, the search for pathological details should be started for this phase of cardiac cycle. Comparing the EP distributions in figure 9.43 with those reconstructed for the healthy subject (figure 9.11), no major differences on the anterior side of the heart can be found. The same observation is true for the TMV distributions (figures 9.45 and 9.13).

The comparison of the posterolateral EP distributions for the patient (figure 9.44) with those for the healthy subject (figure 9.12) reveals a large positive area on the posterior side of the patient's heart, marked in figure 9.44 with arrows. This area is surrounded with a region with negative potential, thus the TMV in this area is lower then that in the surrounded myocardium. This abnormality is not observed for the healthy heart.

The same area remains suspicious in figure 9.46, where the directly reconstructed TMV distributions are shown. Thus a posterior infarction can be assumed. It corresponds to the clinical diagnosis for this patient (see table 6.1).

The second, posterolateral infarction could not be observed, as the lateral wall does not seem to be affected.

The reconstruction of equivalent cardiac sources during the depolarization phase does not deliver reliable results, the correlation is quite low. Still a positive change of EP can be observed on the posterior side of the patient's heart relatively to the healthy subject (see figures 9.39 vs. 9.7) at the end of the QRS complex. This supports the assumption of a posterior infarction.

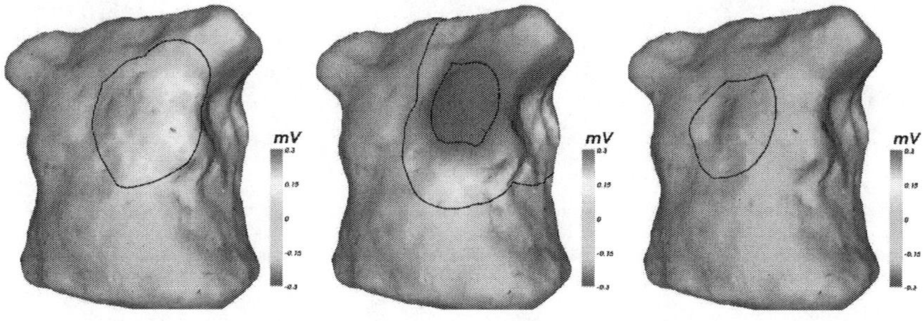

Figure 9.37: *Patient 2. Body surface potential maps (BSPM) during the QRS-complex.*

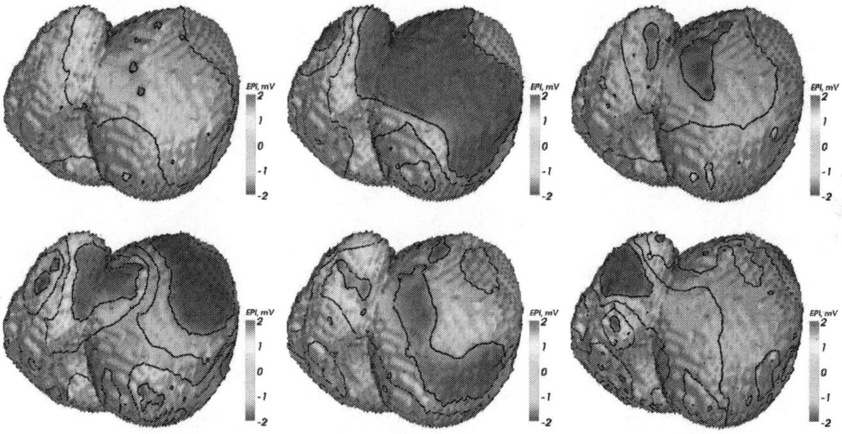

Figure 9.38: *Distributions of EP reconstructed from the measured BSPMs using GMRes (top) as well as TG0 (bottom) regularizations shown in anterior view.*

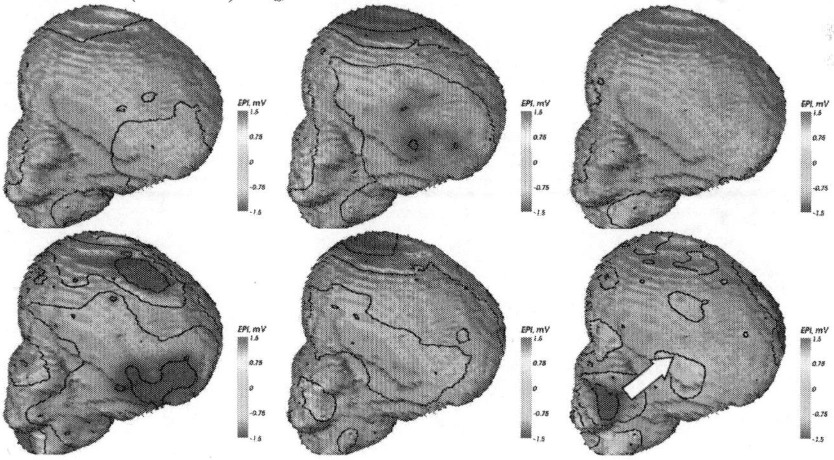

Figure 9.39: *Distributions of EP reconstructed from the measured BSPMs using GMRes (top) as well as TG0 (bottom) regularizations observed from posterolateral direction.*

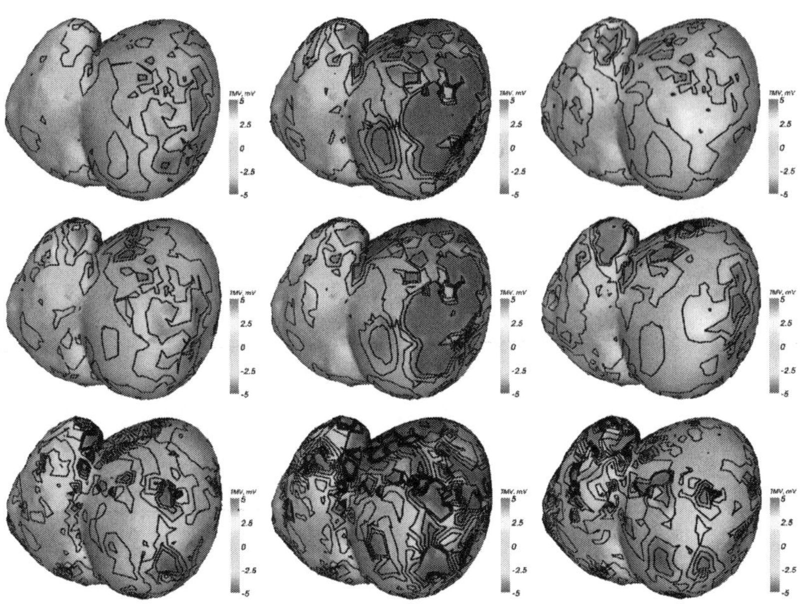

Figure 9.40: *The change of TMV distributions reconstructed from the measured BSPMs using GMRes (top), TG0 (middle) as well as TG2 (bottom) regularizations during the QRS-complex. Anterior view.*

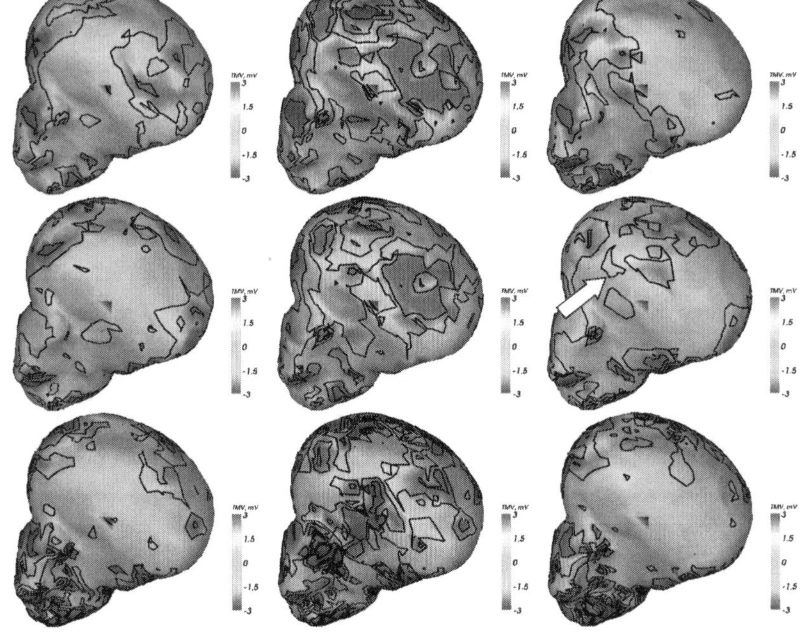

Figure 9.41: *The change of TMV distributions reconstructed from the measured BSPMs using GMRes (top), TG0 (middle) as well as TG2 (bottom) regularizations during the QRS-complex. Posterolateral view.*

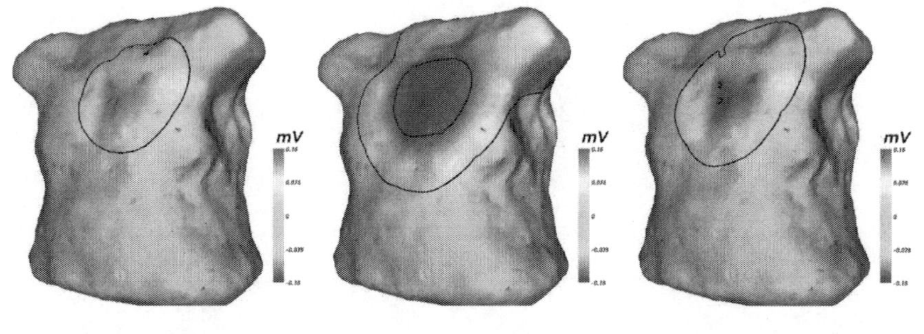

Figure 9.42: *Patient 2. The change of BSPM during the T-wave.*

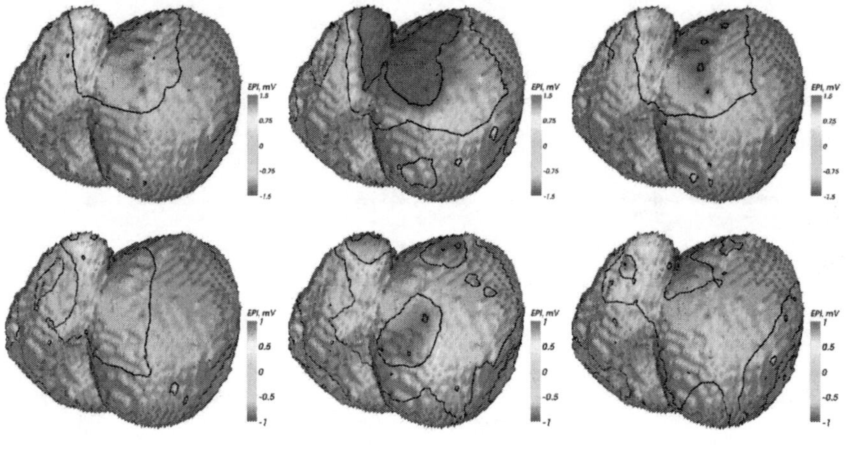

Figure 9.43: *Distributions of EP reconstructed from the measured BSPMs using GMRes regularization (top) as well as TG0 regularization (bottom) during the T-wave. Anterior view.*

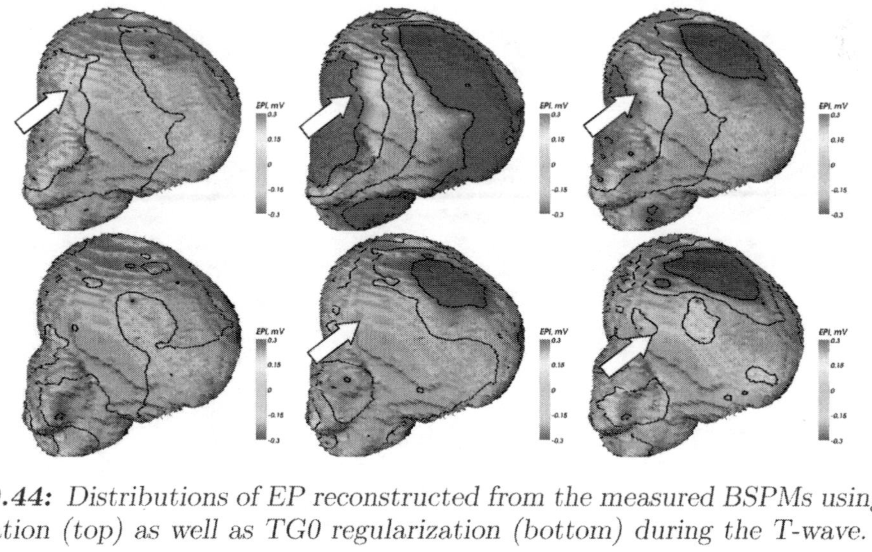

Figure 9.44: *Distributions of EP reconstructed from the measured BSPMs using GMRes regularization (top) as well as TG0 regularization (bottom) during the T-wave. Postero-lateral view.*

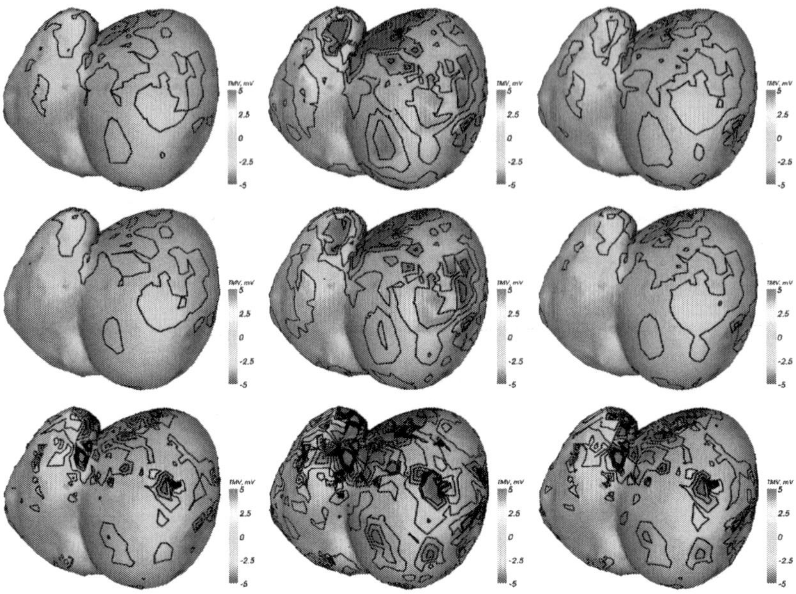

Figure 9.45: *Distributions of TMV reconstructed from the measured BSPMs using GMRes (top), TG0 (middle) as well as TG2 (bottom) regularizations during the T-wave. Anterior view.*

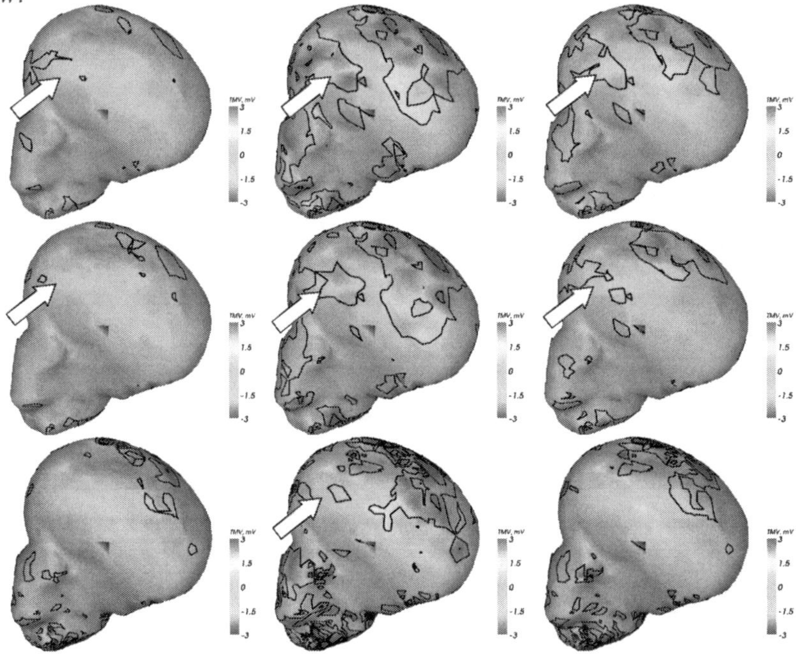

Figure 9.46: *Distributions of TMV reconstructed from the measured BSPMs using GMRes (top), TG0 (middle) as well as TG2 (bottom) regularizations during the T-wave. Posterolateral view.*

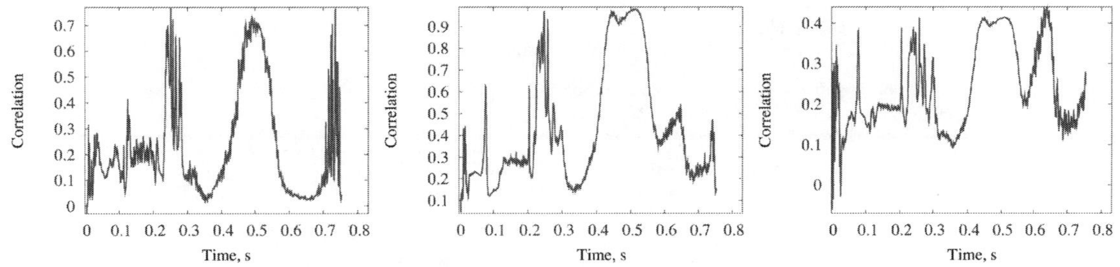

Figure 9.47: *Patient 2. Correlation between the reconstructed EP using GMRes vs. TG0 regularizations (left); between TMV distributions using GMRes vs. TG0 regularizations (middle); using TG2 vs. TG0 regularizations (right).*

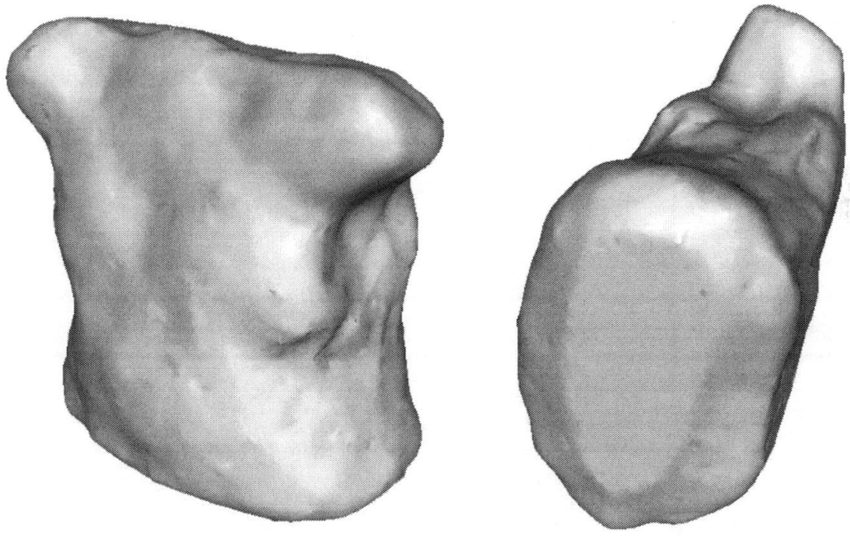

Figure 9.48: *Patient 2. Thorax orientation corresponding to that of the heart: anterior view (left), posterolateral view (right).*

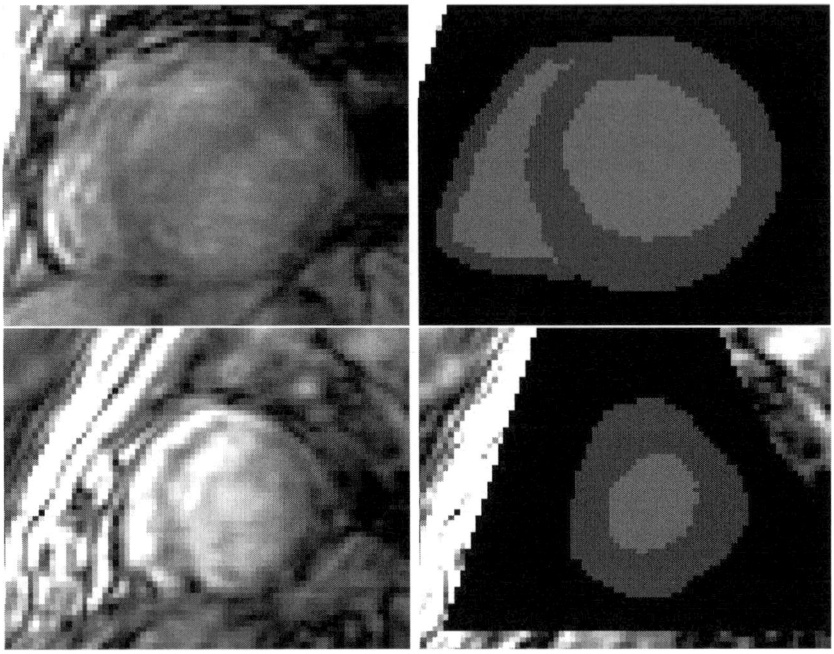

Figure 9.49: *Patient 3. Results of segmentation of the subject's heart (right) compared with the original SAX MRI data set (left). Top: near the ventricular base; bottom: near the apex.*

9.5 Patient 3

9.5.1 Description of the Patient and Segmentation Results

Patient 3, H.S., male, age 43, dilative cardiomyopathy caused by myocarditis was diagnosed. The SAX MR-image of the heart was provided with the resolution of $2.27 \times 2.27 \times 5.5$ mm^3. The image of the thorax had the resolution of $4 \times 4 \times 5$ mm^3.

Figure 9.49 shows the anatomical model of the heart compared with the original MRI data set. The segmentation of the patient's thorax is demonstrated in figure 9.50.

The resulting model of the patient's heart possesses the resolution of $1 \times 1 \times 1$ mm^3 and contains 579,237 excitable voxels. The atria has not been segmented, a region filled up with blood has been created instead in order to obtain a similar distribution of conductivity.

Due to the dilation of the heart a finite element mesh has been created with a relatively large number of nodes: 141,595 nodes and 860,735 tetrahedra. In this way the average distance between nodes within myocardium is sustained at 2 mm. The resulting volume conductor contains heart, lungs, liver, muscles and fat (see figure 9.50).

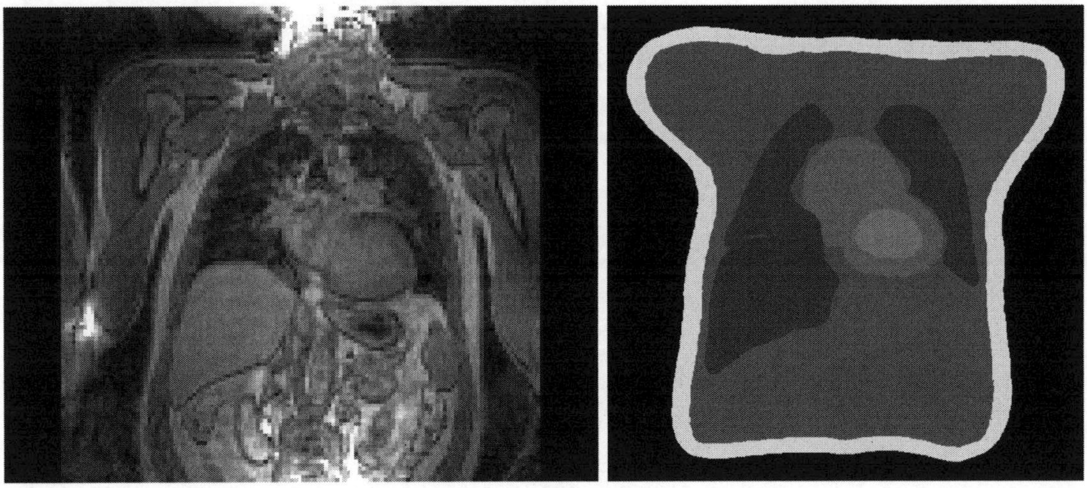

Figure 9.50: *Patient 3. Anatomical model of the subject's thorax (right) compared with the original data set (left).*

9.5.2 Measurement of BSPM

The 64-channel BSPM was recorded during 200 s, with the sample rate of 2048 Hz. In each channel single heart cycles were cut out, superimposed and averaged as described in section 6.3. The resulting ECG is shown in figure 9.51. Dotted vertical lines mark the time points, at which the BSPMs and reconstruction results are shown.

Figure 9.52 demonstrates 12 standard leads obtained from the multichannel ECG measurement. As there was no electrode near the V3 Wilson lead location, this lead was not built.

The ECG is characterized by a large duration of the QRS-complex (about 180 ms) due to the dilation of ventricles. The ST-segment offset is significant.

The potential distributions on the thorax surface during the QRS-complex are shown in figure 9.53, during the T-wave – in figure 9.53. The color scale covers the range between -0.5 and +0.5 mV for the QRS-complex and from -0.3 to +0.3 mV for the T-wave.

9.5.3 Reconstruction Results

The results of EP and TMV reconstructions are shown in figures 9.54-9.62. Table 9.1 contains short descriptions, color ranges as well as the values for equipotential lines used for these figures.

Figure 9.63 represents the correlation between the distributions of EP and TMV obtained using different regularization techniques. The correlation between the EP distributions reconstructed with GMRes and TG0 regularization is high (about 0.9) during both the QRS-complex and T-wave. The TMV distributions resulting from GMRes and TG0 are quite near during the T-wave and at the end of the QRS-complex. The results obtained

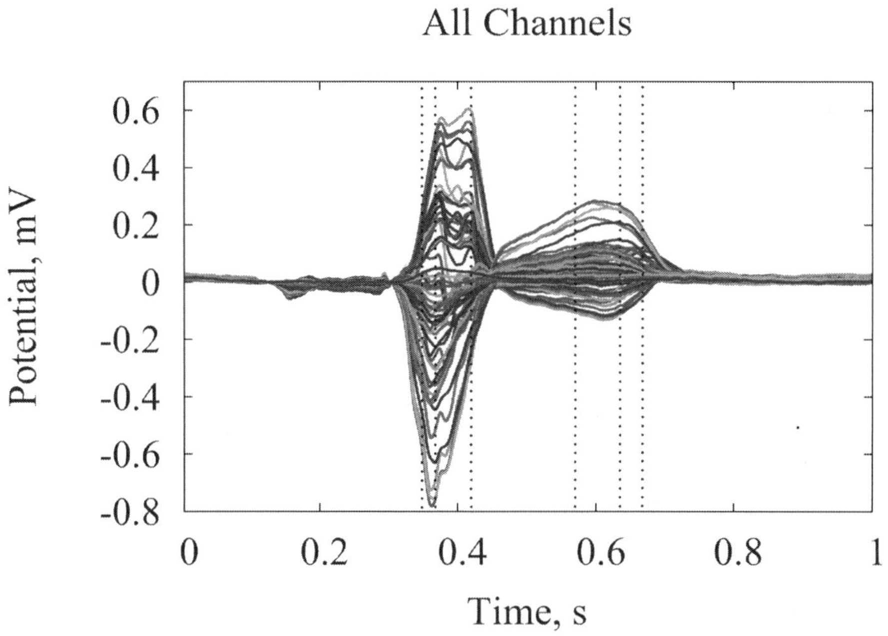

Figure 9.51: *Patient 3. ECG recorded with 64 measurement electrodes. Vertical dotted lines represent the time points at which the reconstruction was performed.*

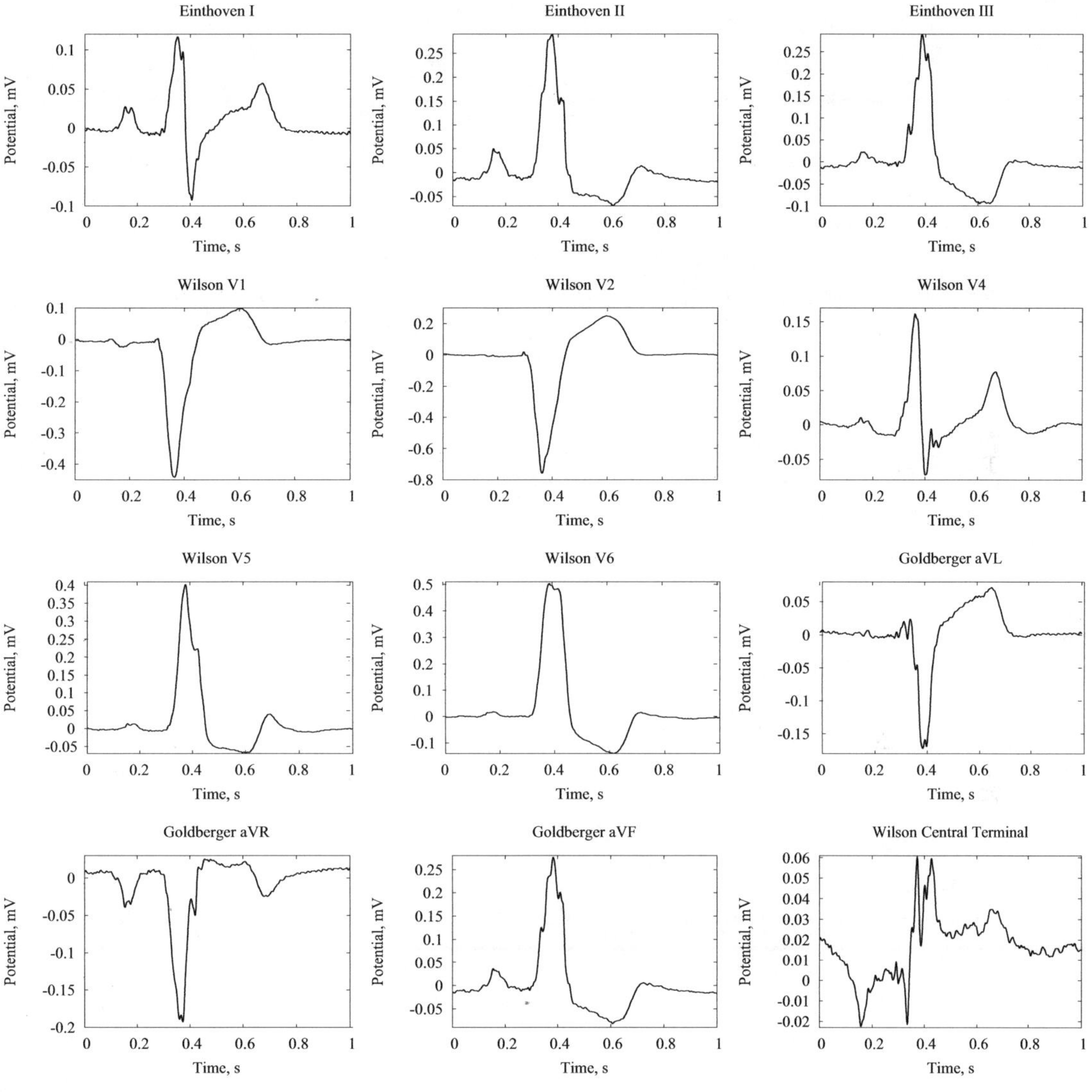

Figure 9.52: *Patient 3. Locations of the standard leads; 64-channel ECG; standard leads. There was no lead among the electrodes near enough to the standard electrode location V3.*

Figure	Description	Color Range	Equipotential Lines
9.53	BSPM during QRS	-0.5..+0.5	-0.45, -0.15, +0.15, +0.45
9.54	EP during QRS anterior	-2..+2	-1.5, -0.5, +0.5, +1.5
9.55	EP during QRS posterior	-2..+2	-1.5, -0.5, +0.5, +1.5
9.56	TMV during QRS anterior	-5..+5	-5, -3, -1, +1, +3, +5
9.57	TMV during QRS posterior	-5..+5	-5, -3, -1, +1, +3, +5
9.58	BSPM during T-wave	-0.3..+0.3	-0.3, -0.1, +0.1, +0.3
9.59	EP during T-wave anterior	-2..+2	-1.5, -0.5, +0.5, +1.5
9.60	EP during T-wave posterior	-2..+2	-1.5, -0.5, +0.5, +1.5
9.61	TMV during T-wave anterior	-5..+5	-5, -3, -1, +1, +3, +5
9.62	TMV during T-wave posterior	-5..+5	-5, -3, -1, +1, +3, +5

Table 9.1: *A short description, color range in mV, equipotential line values in mV for each of the figures representing the reconstruction results for patient 3.*

using TG2 are obviously overregularized.

In figure 9.64 the orientations of thorax corresponding to the anterior and posterolateral views of the heart are shown.

9.5.4 Conclusions

The excitation conduction velocity of the left ventricular myocardium is significantly decreased for this patient. Comparing the three time instants of the QRS-complex shown in figures 9.54 for epicardial potentials and 9.56, a clear drift of the excitation front towards the lateral wall of the left ventricle can be observed. Although the posterior distributions of EP and TMV (figures 9.55 and 9.57, respectively) are very smooth, the same tendency can be observed as well.

The repolarization sequence is clearly the same: the repolarized area, which has a lower TMV and higher EP, is obviously growing towards the lateral side of the left ventricle, whereas for a normal heart the excitation and relaxation sequences are nearly opposite. This can be seen directly in figure 9.52 containing the standard leads of ECG: the QRS-complex and the T-wave have almost everywhere opposite polarities, whereas for the healthy subject (figure 9.4) they are equally polarized.

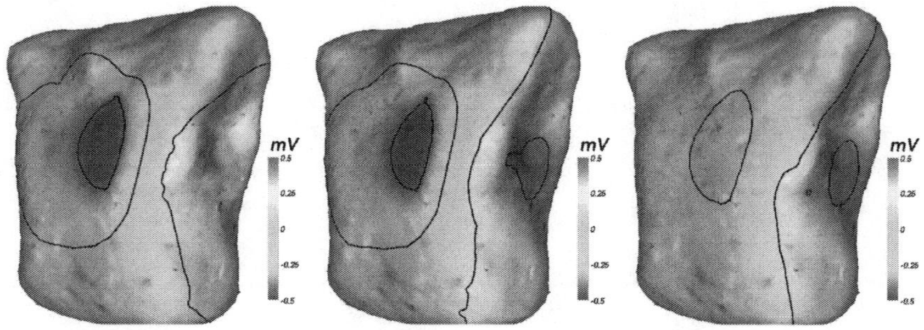

Figure 9.53: *Patient 3. Body surface potential maps (BSPM) during the QRS-complex. Time points are indicated in figure 9.51.*

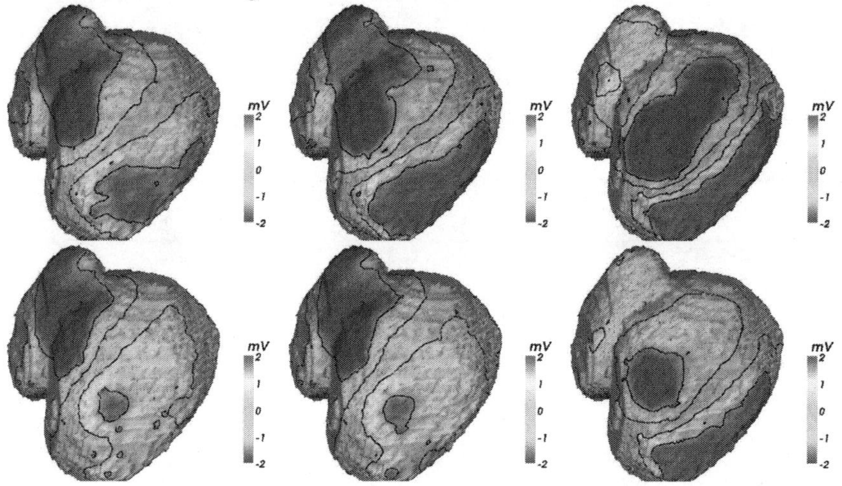

Figure 9.54: *Distributions of EP reconstructed from the measured BSPMs using GMRes (top) as well as TG0 (bottom) regularizations during the QRS-complex shown in anterior view.*

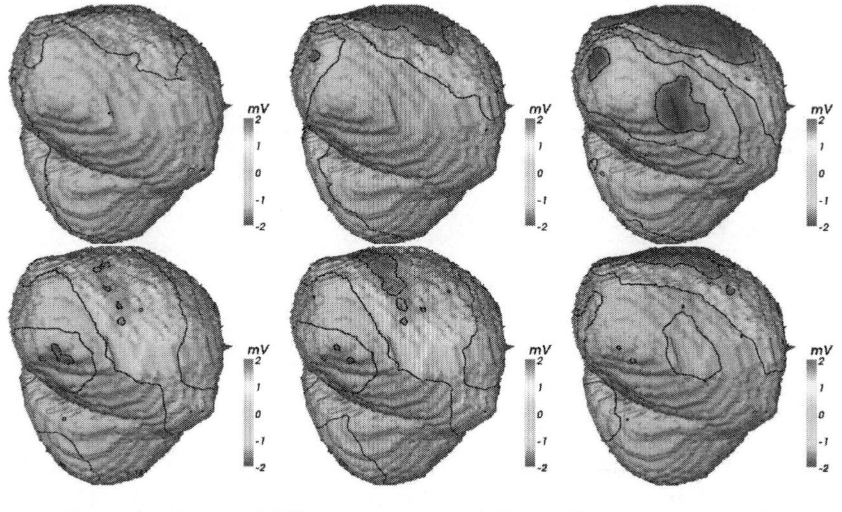

Figure 9.55: *Distributions of EP reconstructed from the measured BSPMs using GM-Res (top) as well as TG0 (bottom) regularizations during the QRS-complex shown from posterolateral direction.*

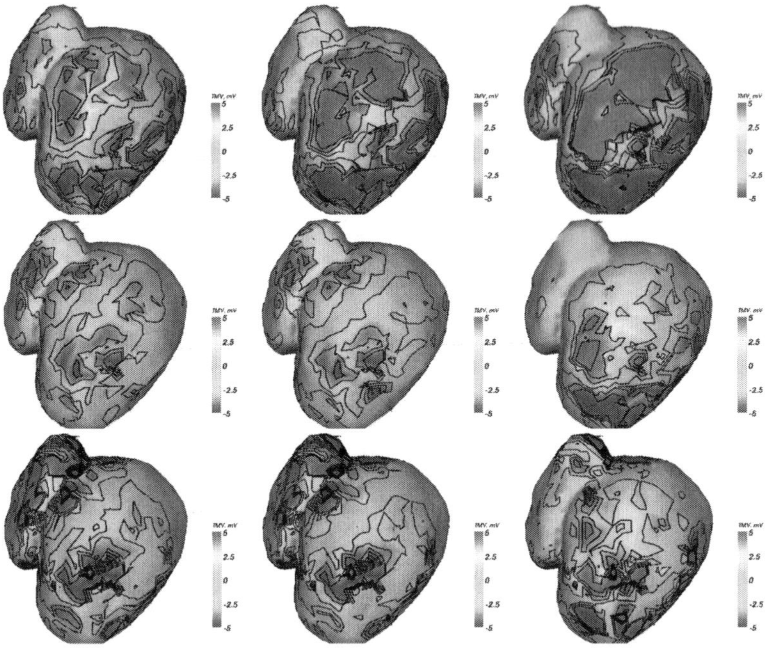

Figure 9.56: *Distributions of TMV reconstructed from the measured BSPMs using GM-Res (top), TG0 (middle) as well as TG2 (bottom) regularizations during the QRS-complex shown in anterior view.*

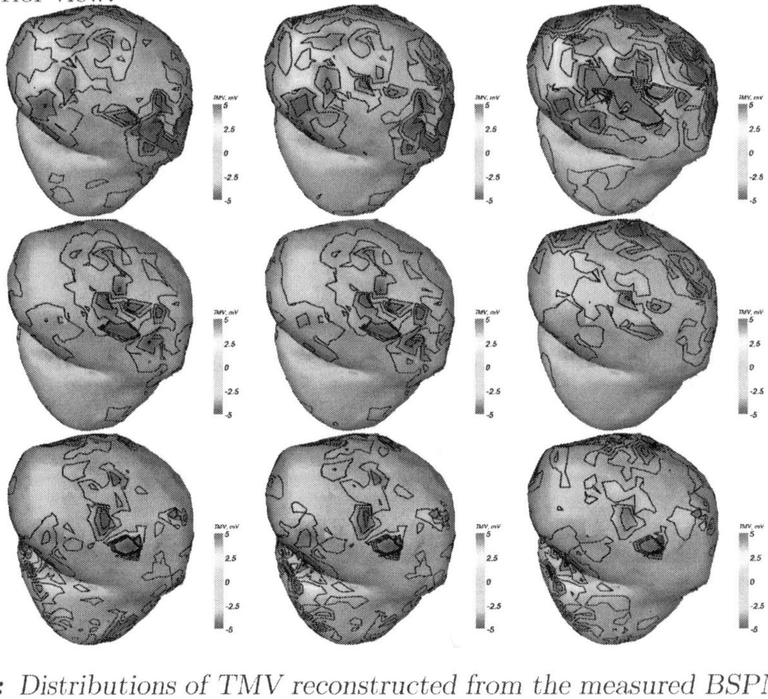

Figure 9.57: *Distributions of TMV reconstructed from the measured BSPMs using GM-Res (top), TG0 (middle) as well as TG2 (bottom) regularizations during the QRS-complex. Posterolateral view.*

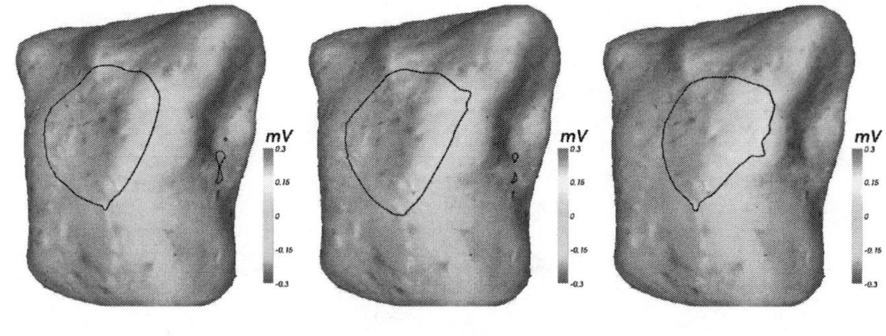

Figure 9.58: *Patient 3. BSPM during the T-wave.*

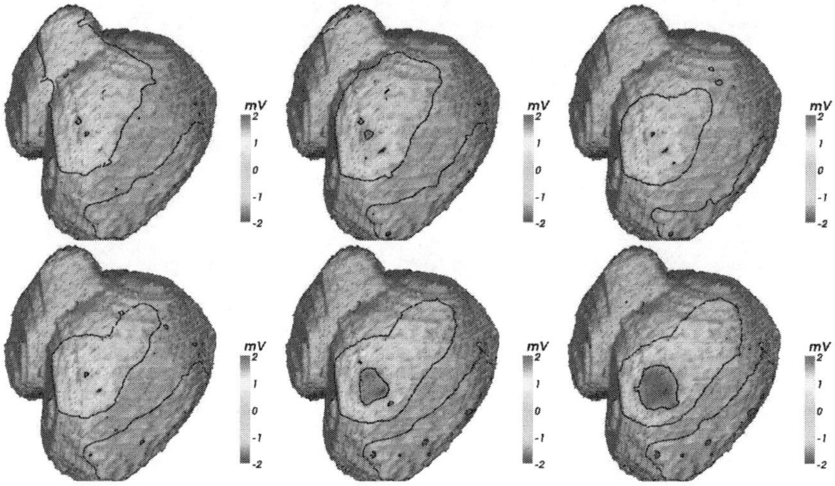

Figure 9.59: *Distributions of EP reconstructed from the measured BSPMs using GMRes regularization (top) as well as TG0 regularization (bottom) during the T-wave shown in anterior view.*

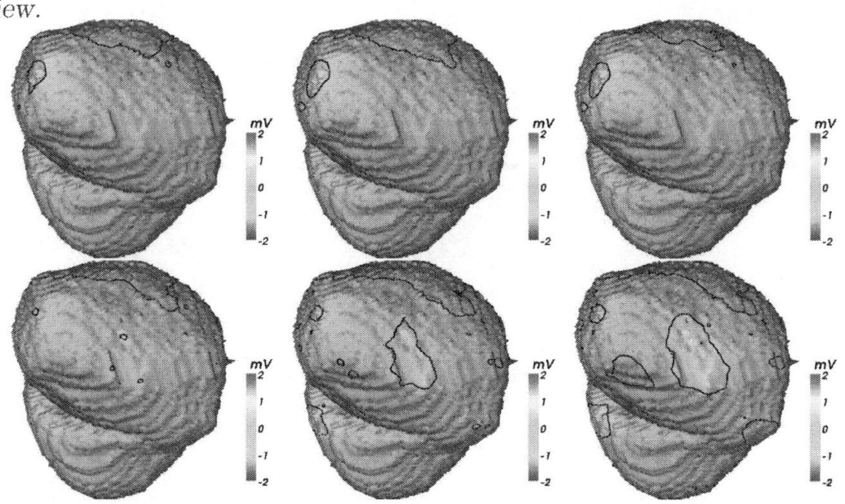

Figure 9.60: *Distributions of EP reconstructed from the measured BSPMs using GMRes regularization (top) as well as TG0 regularization (bottom) during the T-wave. Postero-lateral view.*

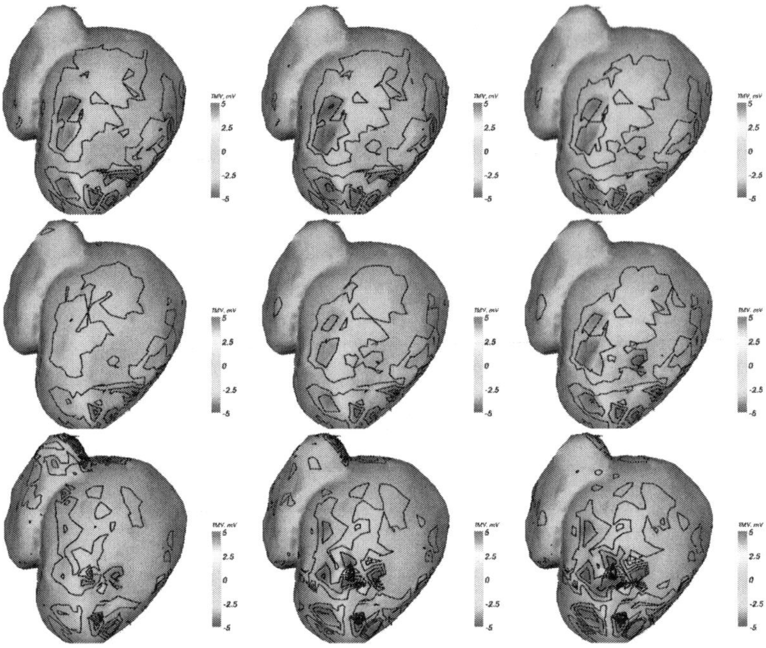

Figure 9.61: *Distributions of TMV reconstructed from the measured BSPMs using GM-Res (top), TG0 (middle) as well as TG2 (bottom) regularizations during the T-wave shown in anterior view.*

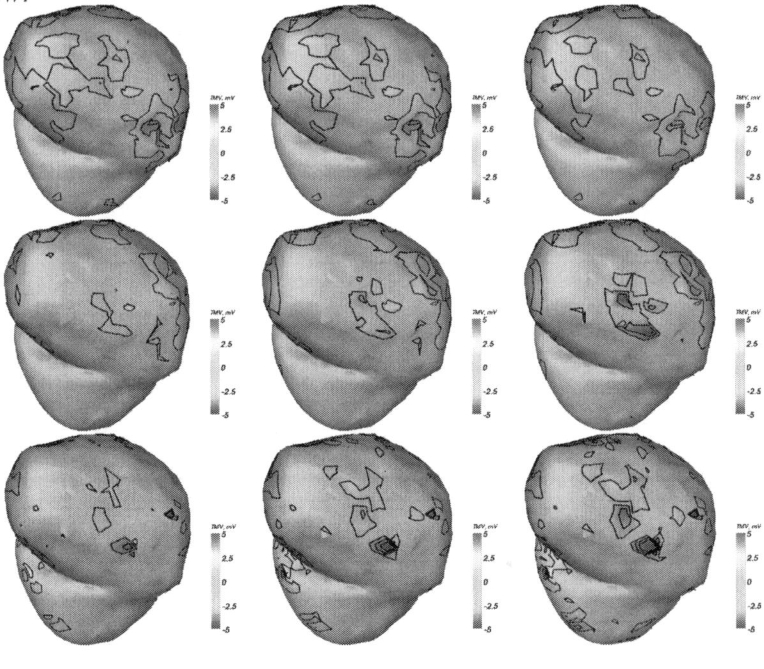

Figure 9.62: *Distributions of TMV reconstructed from the measured BSPMs using GM-Res (top), TG0 (middle) as well as TG2 (bottom) regularizations during the T-wave. Posterolateral view.*

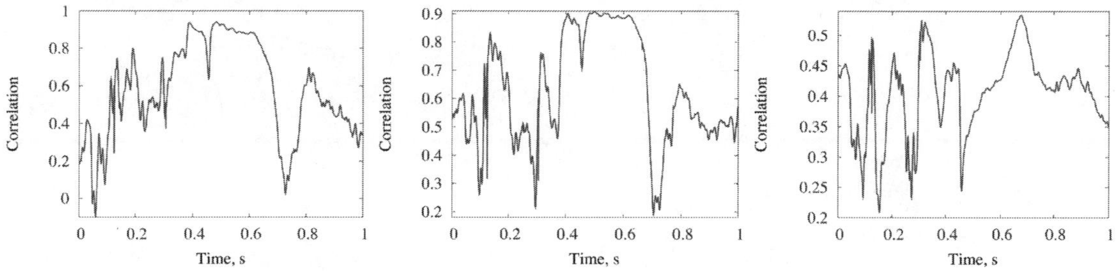

Figure 9.63: *Patient 3. Correlation between the reconstructed EP using GMRes vs. TG0 regularizations (left); between TMV distributions using GMRes vs. TG0 regularizations (middle); using TG2 vs. TG0 regularizations (right).*

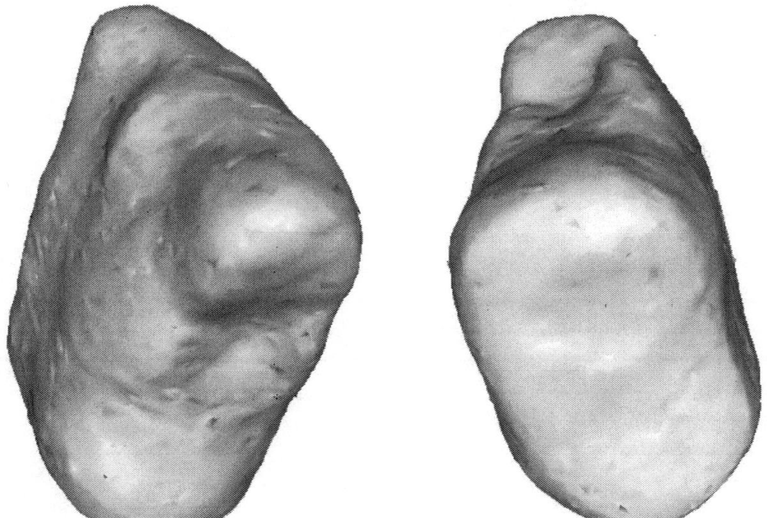

Figure 9.64: *Patient 3. Thorax orientation corresponding to that of the heart: anterior view (left), posterolateral view (right).*

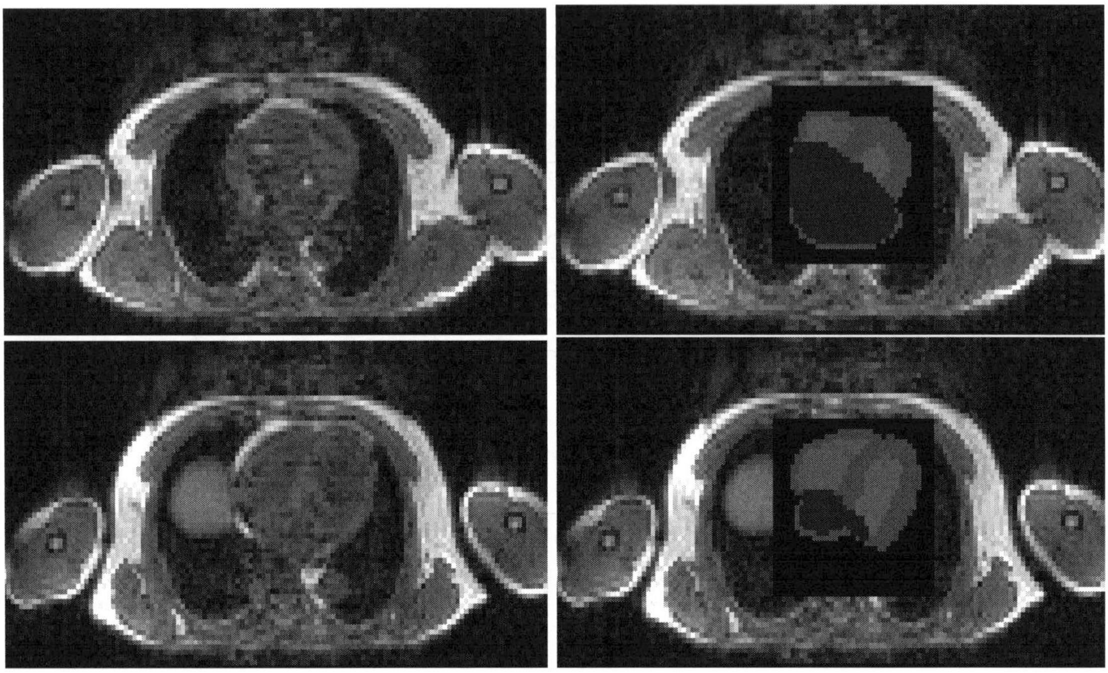

Figure 9.65: Patient 4. Results of segmentation of the subject's heart (right) compared with the original SAX MRI data set (left). Top: near the ventricular base; bottom: near the apex.

9.6 Patient 4

9.6.1 Description of the Patient and Segmentation Results

Patient 4, P.H., male, age 54, a new anterior infarction is diagnosed. Resolution of the heart MRI data set is $2.27 \times 2.27 \times 4\ mm^3$, thorax – $4 \times 4 \times 4.69\ mm^3$. Merging problems were experienced during the segmentation of these data sets, as their global coordinate systems did not match. Thus the resulting heart model had to be "shifted" in order to fit into the thorax. The segmentation of the heart is shown in figure 9.65, that of the thorax in figure 9.66.

Another cardiac MRI data set has been made with a contrast agent (gadolinium) introduced in order to reveal the location of infarction. In this way the quality of reconstruction can be estimated. Several slices with segmented infarction scar are shown in figure 9.67.

The anatomical model of the heart has been created with the resolution of $1 \times 1 \times 1\ mm^3$ and contains 275,243 excitable voxels. The atria have been segmented schematically.

The finite element model of volume conductor contains 85,390 nodes and 524,539 tetrahedra. The average distance between nodes in ventricular myocardium is 2 mm. The model contains lungs, heart, liver, muscles and fat.

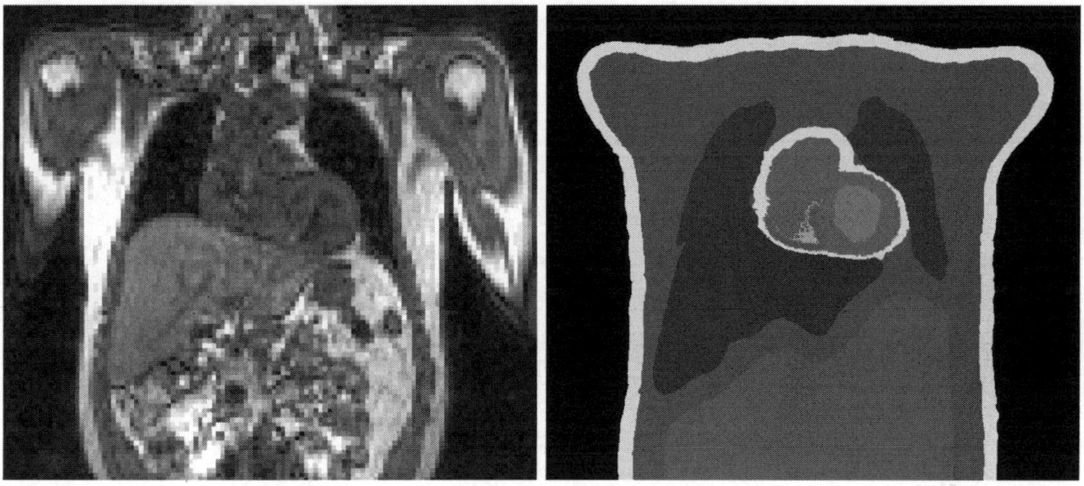

Figure 9.66: *Patient 4. Anatomical model of the subject's thorax (right) compared with the original data set (left).*

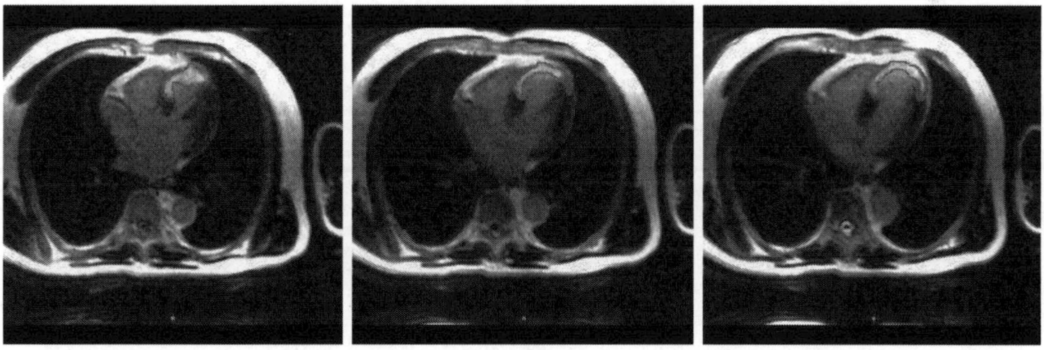

Figure 9.67: *Patient 4. MRI images of the heart with the infarction scar revealed using a contrast agent (gadolinium).*

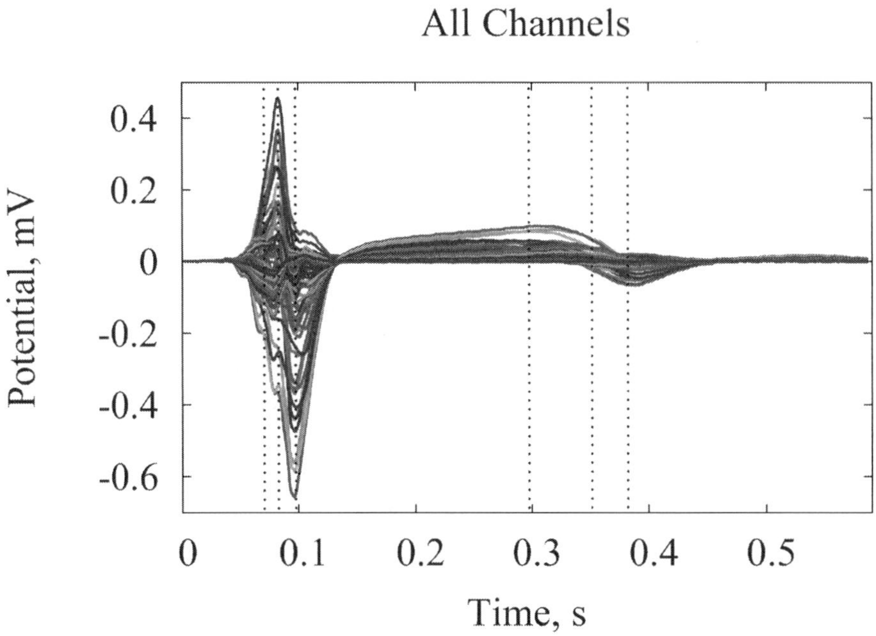

Figure 9.68: *Patient 4. ECG recorded with 64 measurement electrodes. Vertical dotted lines represent the time points at which the reconstruction was performed.*

9.6.2 Measurement of BSPM

The 64-channel ECG was recorded with the BioSemi system. The sample rate was set to 2048 Hz. The ECG was recorded during 200 s, single ECG cycles were cut out, superimposed and averaged as described in section 6.3. The resulting set of ECG curves including the QRS-complex and T-wave is shown in figure 9.68.

Figure 9.69 shows the standard leads of the measured ECG. As there was no electrode located near enough to the standard location of V1, the corresponding ECG lead is not shown.

BSPMs at the beginning, in the middle and at the end of the QRS complex is shown in figure 9.70. The potential distributions on the body surface during the ST-segment and T-wave are shown in figure 9.75. The corresponding time points are marked in figure 9.68.

9.6.3 Reconstruction Results: Tikhonov-Greensite, GMRes

The distributions of epicardial potentials and transmembrane voltages for patient 4 are shown in figures 9.71-9.79. Table 9.2 contains the information about these figures such as short descriptions, color scales and the values at which the isolines are shown. The distributions of TMV during the T-wave obtained using the GMRes regularization have a smaller amplitude, so different color scales have been chosen.

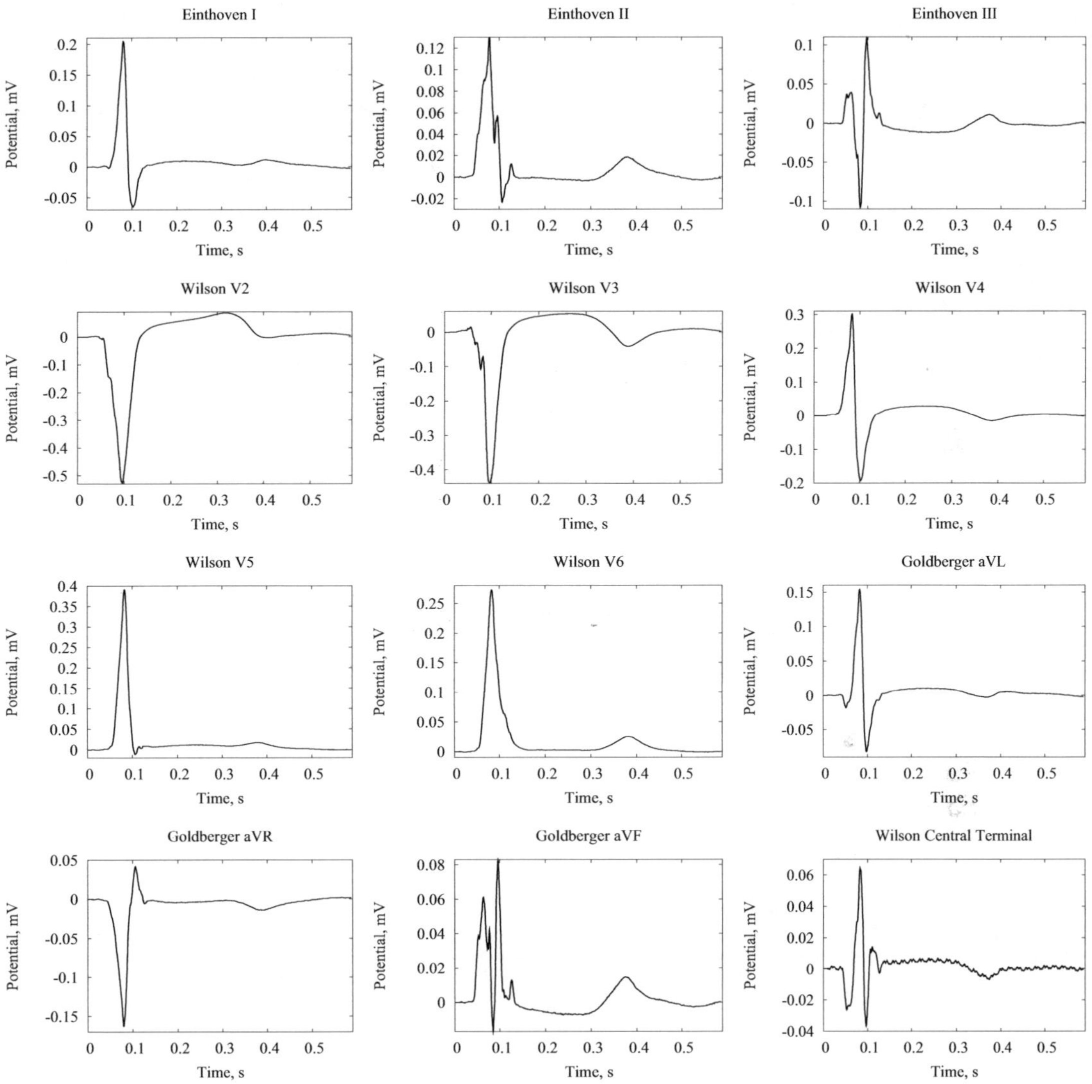

Figure 9.69: *Patient 4. Locations of the standard leads; 64-channel ECG; standard leads. There was no lead among the electrodes near enough to the standard electrode location V1.*

Figure	Description	Color Range	Equipotential Lines
9.70	BSPM during QRS	-0.3..+0.3	-0.3, -0.1, +0.1, +0.3
9.71	EP during QRS anterior	-5..+5	-5, -3, -1, +1, +3, +5
9.72	EP during QRS posterior	-5..+5	-5, -3, -1, +1, +3, +5
9.73	TMV during QRS anterior	-10..+10	-10, -6, -2, +2, +6, +10
9.74	TMV during QRS posterior	-10..+10	-10, -6, -2, +2, +6, +10
9.75	BSPM during T-wave	-0.05..+0.05	-0.05, -0.03, ..., +0.05
9.76	EP during T-wave anterior	-1.5..+1.5	-1.5, -0.5, +0.5, +1.5
9.77	EP during T-wave posterior	-1.5..+1.5	-1.5, -0.5, +0.5, +1.5
9.78	TMV during T-wave anterior	-5(-3)..(+3)+5	(-5,) -3, -1, +1, +3(, +5)
9.79	TMV during T-wave posterior	-5(-3)..(+3)+5	(-5,) -3, -1, +1, +3(, +5)

Table 9.2: *A short description, color range in mV, equipotential line values in mV for each of the figures representing the reconstruction results for patient 4. The distributions of TMV during the T-wave are shown with a smaller color range for GMRes than for other regularization methods*

Figure 9.80 represents the change of correlation between the cardiac sources computed with different regularization techniques. The reconstruction of epicardial potentials results in the correlation of about 0.9 during the whole heart cycle. TMV is reconstructed with a worse quality.

The orientation of thorax corresponding to that of the heart in anterior and postero-lateral views is shown in figure 9.81.

9.6.4 Reconstruction Results: MAP-Regularization

As the exact location and size of infarction scar for this patient is known from late enhancement MRI data set, it is interesting to try out the *maximum a posteriori* regularization. In order to perform this computation, the following steps have been made.

First, a statistical basis has been created using the cellular automaton based cardiac model. This basis includes the simulation results (containing transmembrane voltage distributions, potential distributions for the whole thorax as well as simulated ECG) for 60 different configurations of infarction scar. Considered have been 10 infarction locations (1 apical, 4 around the apex and 5 around the basis of the left ventricle), 2 sizes (40 and 60 mm) and 3 depths (located mostly at endocardium, midmyocardium or epicardium). The development of such basis has been described in section 8.4 in more detail.

Second, a compound vector of 7 sequential TMV distributions during the ST-segment has been created for each configuration of infarction scar, as described in subsection 5.3.5. The covariance matrix of *a priori* estimations C_x has been computed out of these vectors. The covariance matrix of noise C_e is assumed to be diagonal and include the estimated size of noise and systematic errors equal to 1 mV^2.

Afterwards the estimator H has been computed and the inverse problem has been solved. The resulting TMV distribution in the middle of the ST-segment is shown in figure

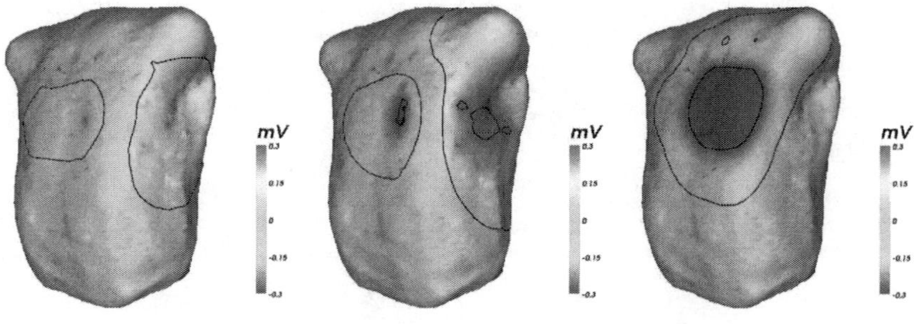

Figure 9.70: *Patient 4. Body surface potential maps (BSPM) during the QRS-complex. The time instants are marked in figure 9.68.*

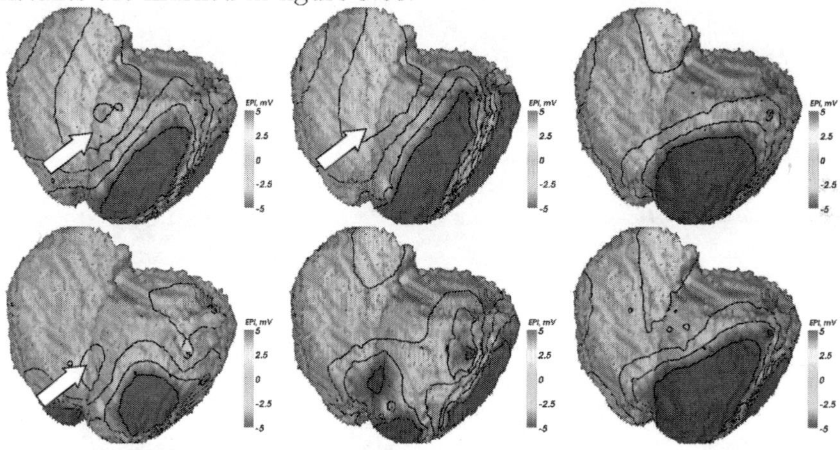

Figure 9.71: *Distributions of EP reconstructed from the measured BSPMs using GMRes (top) as well as TG0 (bottom) regularizations. Anterior view.*

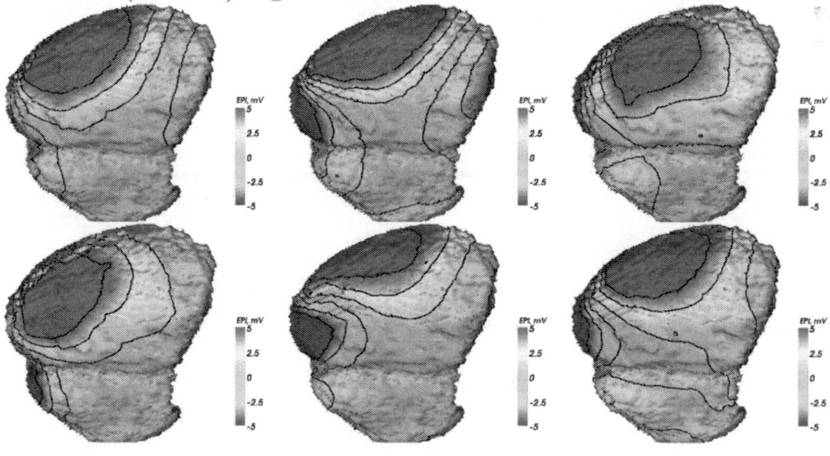

Figure 9.72: *Distributions of EP reconstructed from the measured BSPMs using GMRes (top) as well as TG0 (bottom) regularizations. Posterolateral view.*

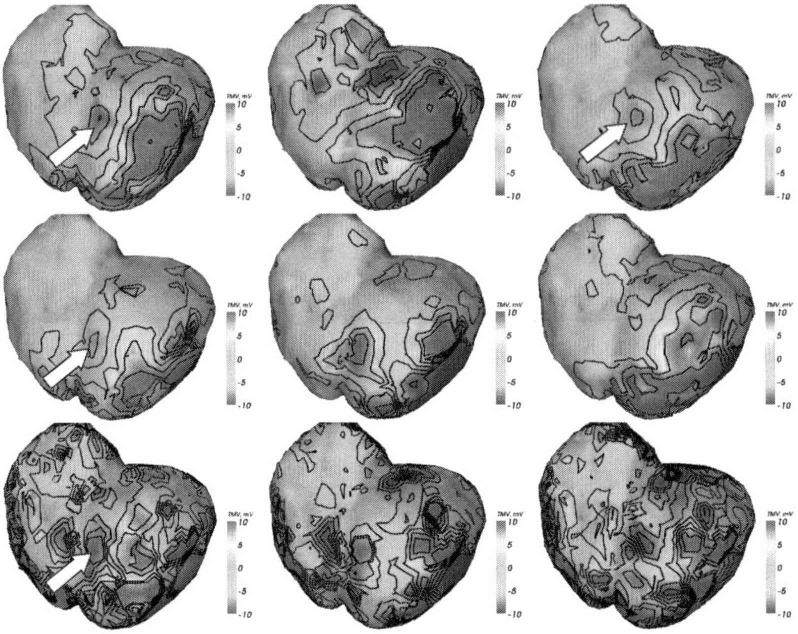

Figure 9.73: *Distributions of TMV reconstructed from the measured BSPMs using GM-Res (top), TG0 (middle) as well as TG2 (bottom) regularizations. Anterior view.*

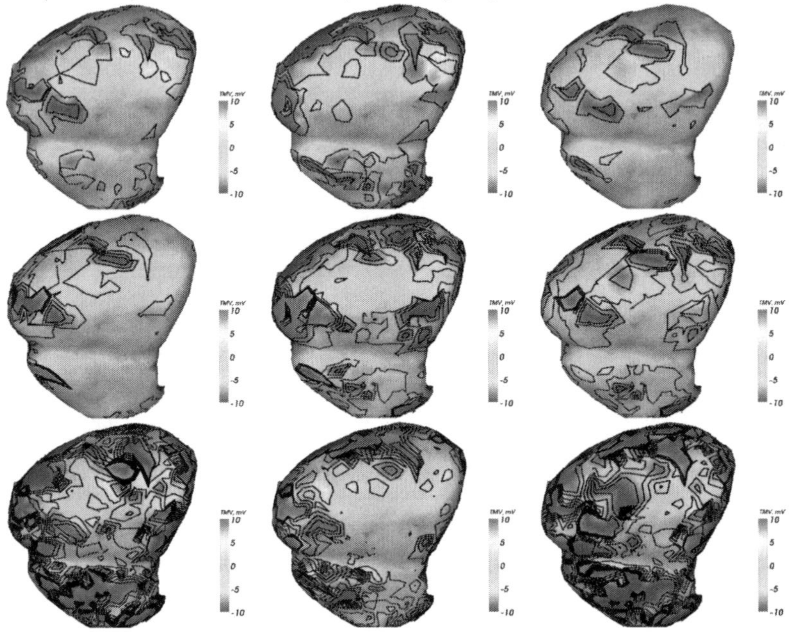

Figure 9.74: *Distributions of TMV reconstructed from the measured BSPMs using GM-Res (top), TG0 (middle) as well as TG2 (bottom) regularizations. Posterolateral view.*

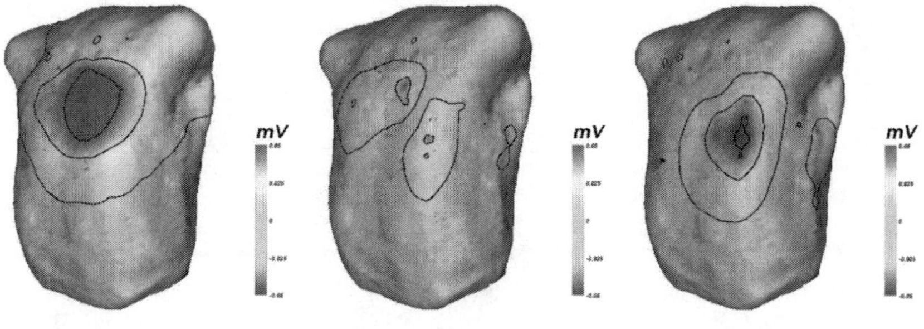

Figure 9.75: *Patient 4. BSPM during the T-wave. Time points* $t = 0.679,\ 0.718,\ 0.757$ *s are shown.*

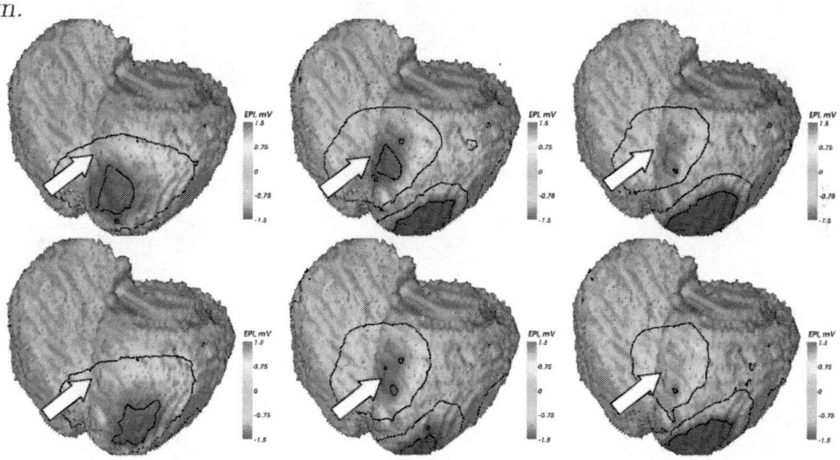

Figure 9.76: *Distributions of EP reconstructed from the measured BSPMs using GMRes regularization (top) as well as TG0 regularization (bottom). Anterior view.*

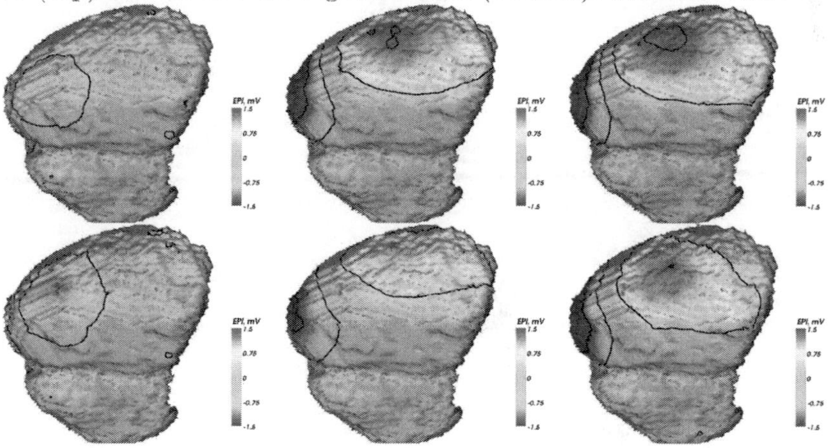

Figure 9.77: *Distributions of EP reconstructed from the measured BSPMs using GMRes regularization (top) as well as TG0 regularization (bottom). Posterolateral view.*

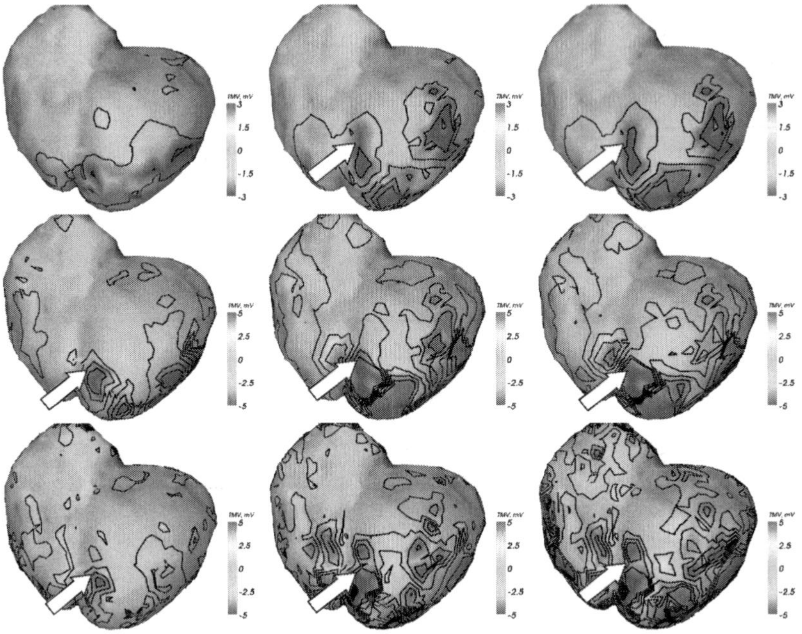

Figure 9.78: *Distributions of TMV reconstructed from the measured BSPMs using GM-Res (top), TG0 (middle) as well as TG2 (bottom) regularizations. Anterior view.*

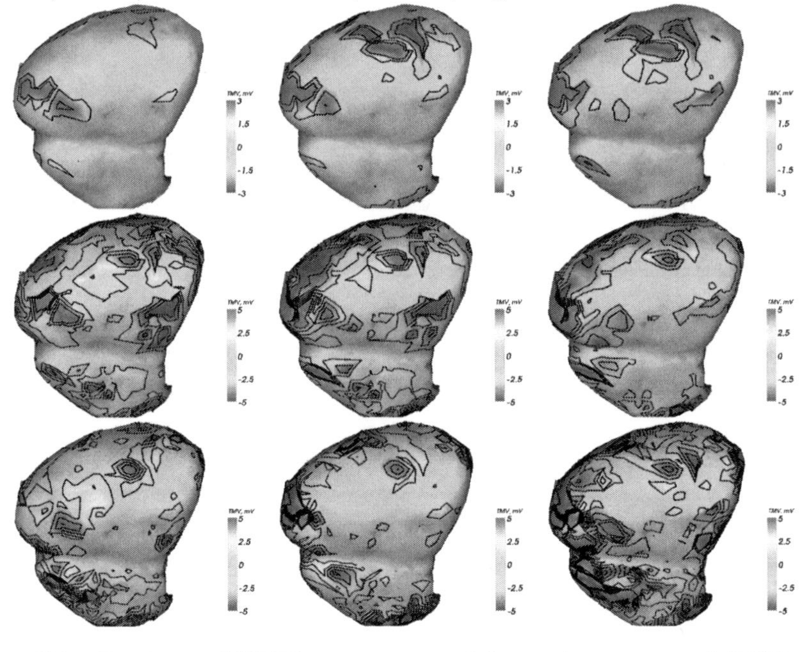

Figure 9.79: *Distributions of TMV reconstructed from the measured BSPMs using GM-Res (top), TG0 (middle) as well as TG2 (bottom) regularizations. Posterolateral view.*

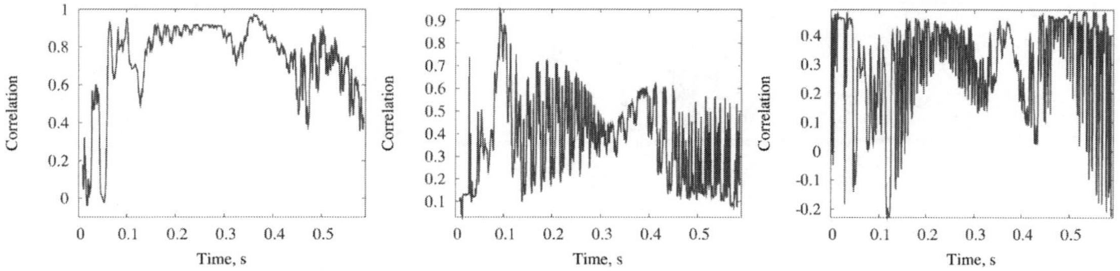

Figure 9.80: *Patient 4. Correlation between the reconstructed EP using GMRes vs. TG0 regularizations (left); between TMV distributions using GMRes vs. TG0 regularizations (middle); using TG2 vs. TG0 regularizations (right).*

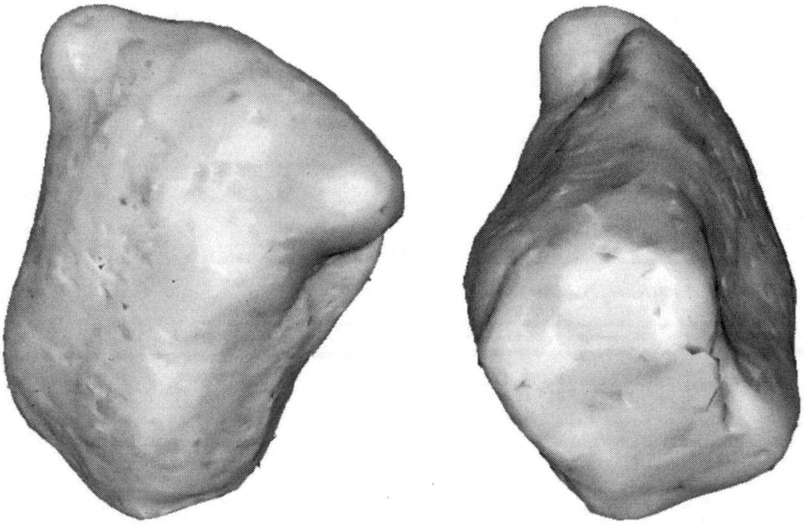

Figure 9.81: *Patient 4. Thorax orientation corresponding to that of the heart: anterior view (left), posterolateral view (right).*

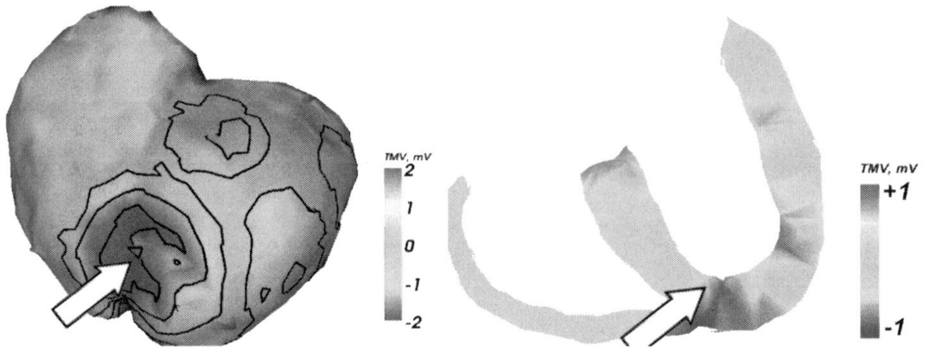

Figure 9.82: *Distribution of transmembrane voltages reconstructed using the spatio-temporal maximum a posteriori regularization method for the middle of the ST-segment. Anterior view of the heart (left) and a transverse cross section (right) are shown.*

9.82.

9.6.5 Conclusions

For this patient the best correlation was between the EP obtained using the GMRes vs. TG0 regularization approaches (see figure 9.80, left). Considering figure 9.71, an area with positive potential (which corresponds to the smaller TMV) surrounded by the regions of negative potential can be distinctly seen at the beginning and (for the GMRes regularization) in the middle of the QRS-complex. This feature can be seen even better when comparing the heart surface potential distributions in figure 9.71 with those of the healthy subject (figure 9.6).

The same abnormality can be seen also in the direct reconstruction of TMV (figure 9.73). It can be explained by a lower excitation conduction velocity and excitation amplitude in the area near the infarction.

In the figures depicting the repolarization of the ventricular myocardium (9.76 for EP, 9.78 for TMV), the same abnormality is clearly visible. The quality of reconstruction is even better, as there are no signals with a high spatial frequency which could be corrupted by regularization.

MAP-based regularization is able to reveal the anterior infarction even more reliably (see figure 9.82). Thus the location of infarction revealed by the solution of the inverse problem corresponds well with the MR-image made with gadolinium for all demonstrated regularization methods.

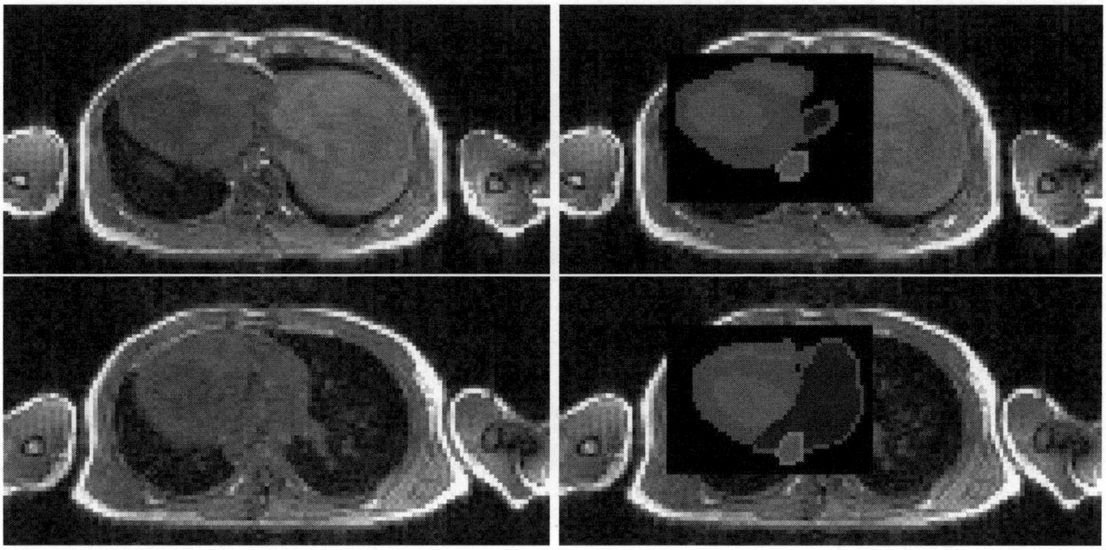

Figure 9.83: *Patient 5. Results of segmentation of the subject's heart (right) compared with the original SAX MRI data set (left). Top: near the ventricular base; bottom: near the apex.*

9.7 Patient 5

9.7.1 Description of the Patient and Segmentation Results

Patient 5, W.O., male, age 46, left bundle branch block is diagnosed. The left ventricle is strongly dilated. Resolution of the heart MRI data set was $1.17 \times 1.17 \times 5.5\ mm^3$, thorax – $4 \times 4 \times 4.69\ mm^3$. The global coordinate systems of these data sets were different, the heart in the cardiac data set was shifted relatively to the heart location in the thoracic data set. Thus after the segmentation of the heart corresponding changes in the transformation matrix had to be done manually. The result of cardiac segmentation is shown in figure 9.83, the volume conductor mesh is compared with the thoracic MRI data set in figure 9.84.

The anatomical model of the heart has the resolution of $1 \times 1 \times 1\ mm^3$ and contains 548,933 excitable voxels. Only schematic segmentation of atria has been performed. The finite element mesh of the volume conductor contains 162,841 nodes and 991,472 tetrahedra. 91,892 nodes are located within the ventricles, with the average distance between nodes being 2 mm. The thorax model contains also lungs, liver, spleen, kidneys, muscles and fat.

9.7.2 Measurement of BSPM

The 64-channel ECG for this patient was recorded during 200 s with the sample rate of 2048 Hz. Also in this case the single ECG cycles in each channel were cut out and superimposed, afterwards the averaging was performed in order to reduce the uncorrelated

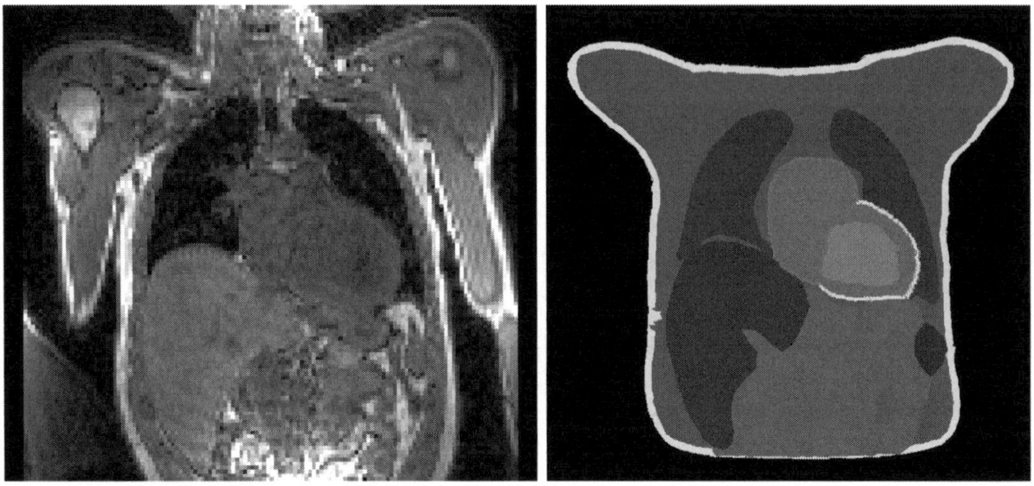

Figure 9.84: *Patient 5. Anatomical model of the subject's thorax (right) compared with the original data set (left).*

noise. The resulting family of 64 ECG signals during a single heart cycle is shown in figure 9.85. Six dotted lines denote the time steps at which the reconstructed distributions of EP and TMV are shown.

The standard leads (all but Wilson V4) are shown in figure 9.86.

The BSPMs interpolated on the whole body surface for the time points marked in figure 9.85 are shown in figures 9.87 (QRS-complex) and 9.92 (T-wave).

9.7.3 Reconstruction Results

Figures 9.88-9.96 show the reconstructed distributions of EP and TMV for patient 5 during the QRS-complex and T-wave, anterior and posterolateral views. Table 9.3 contains short descriptions of these figures, color ranges as well as the values where isolines are shown.

The correlation between the results obtained using different regularization methods is shown in figure 9.97. The quality of EP reconstruction is satisfactory (correlation of about 0.6-0.7) for the whole heart cycle, whereas the correlation between the reconstructed distributions of TMV is quite low.

Figure 9.98 demonstrates the orientation of the thorax corresponding to the anterior and posterolateral views of the heart.

9.7.4 Conclusions

According to figure 9.97, the agreement of TMV distributions obtained with different regularization approaches is quite low because of obvious overregularization, thus the heart surface potentials are to be considered. It can be easily seen in figure 9.88, especially for

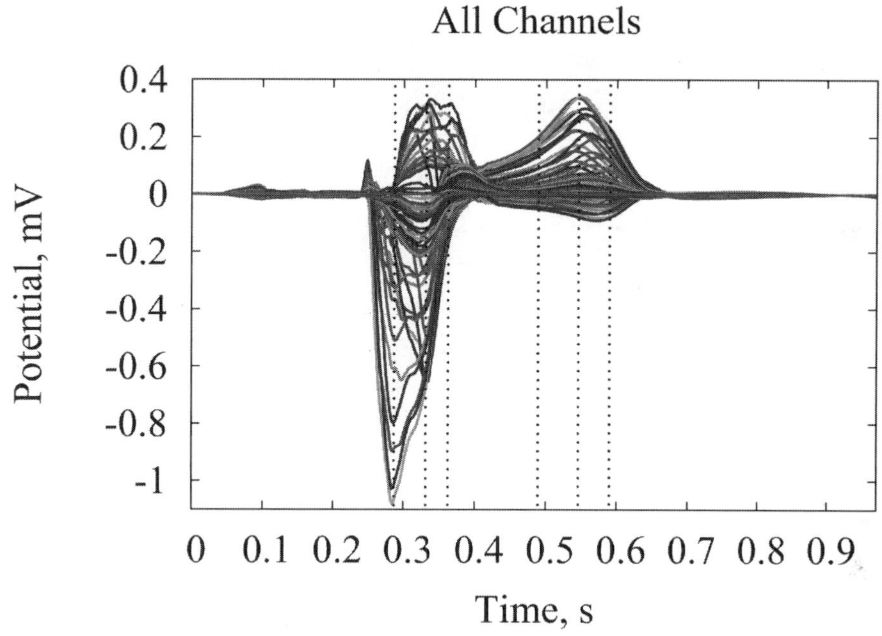

Figure 9.85: *Patient 5. ECG recorded with 64 measurement electrodes. Vertical dotted lines represent the time points at which the reconstruction was performed.*

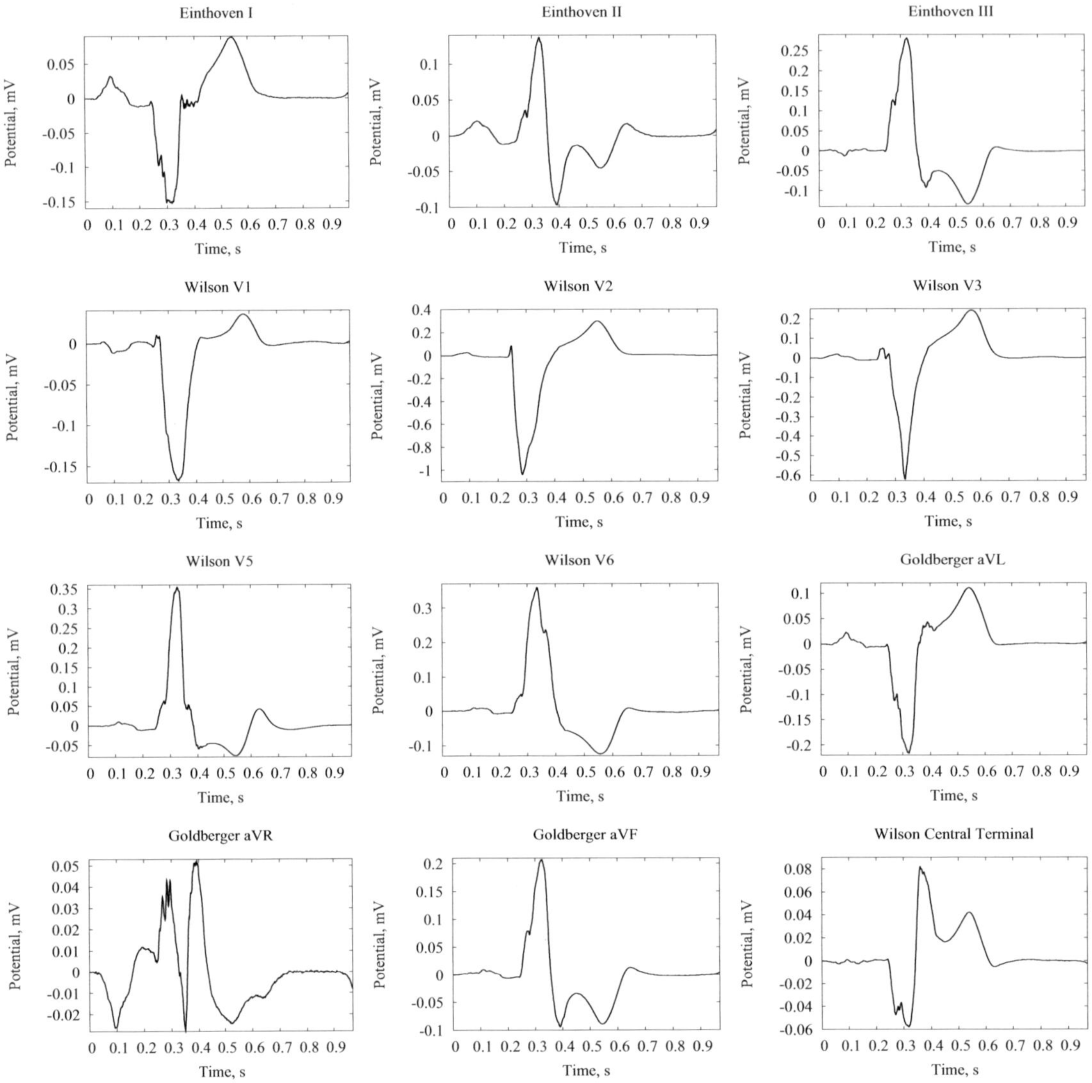

Figure 9.86: *Patient 5. Locations of the standard leads; 64-channel ECG; standard leads. There was no lead among the electrodes near enough to the standard electrode location V4.*

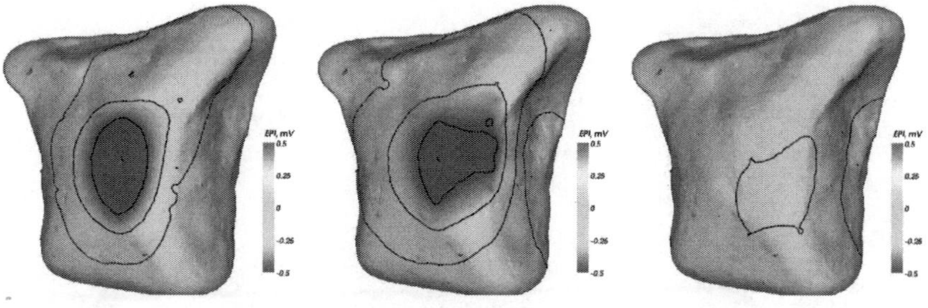

Figure 9.87: *Patient 5. Body surface potential maps (BSPM) during the QRS-complex. Time points are shown in figure 9.85.*

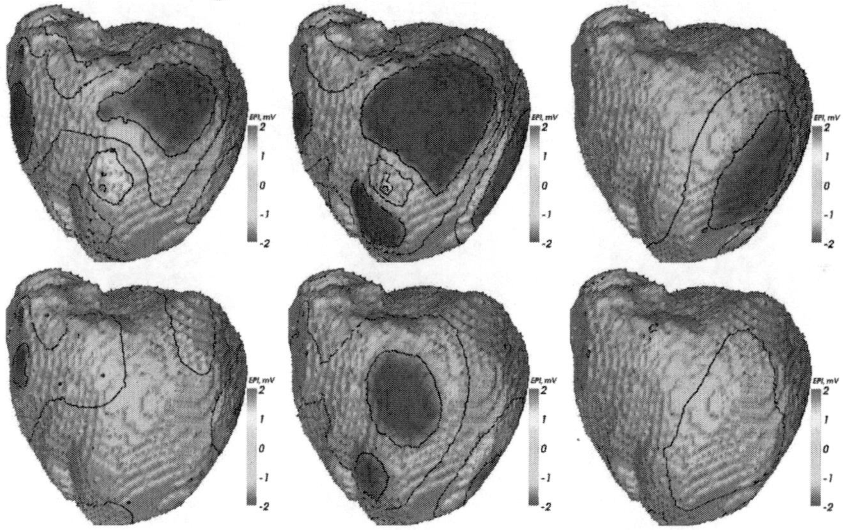

Figure 9.88: *Distributions of EP reconstructed from the measured BSPMs using GMRes (top) as well as TG0 (bottom) regularizations. Anterior view.*

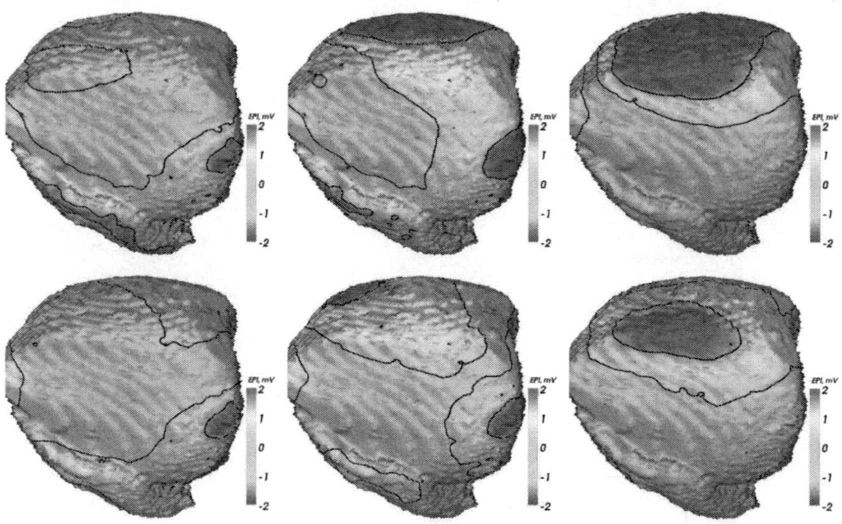

Figure 9.89: *Distributions of EP reconstructed from the measured BSPMs using GMRes (top) as well as TG0 (bottom) regularizations. Posterolateral view.*

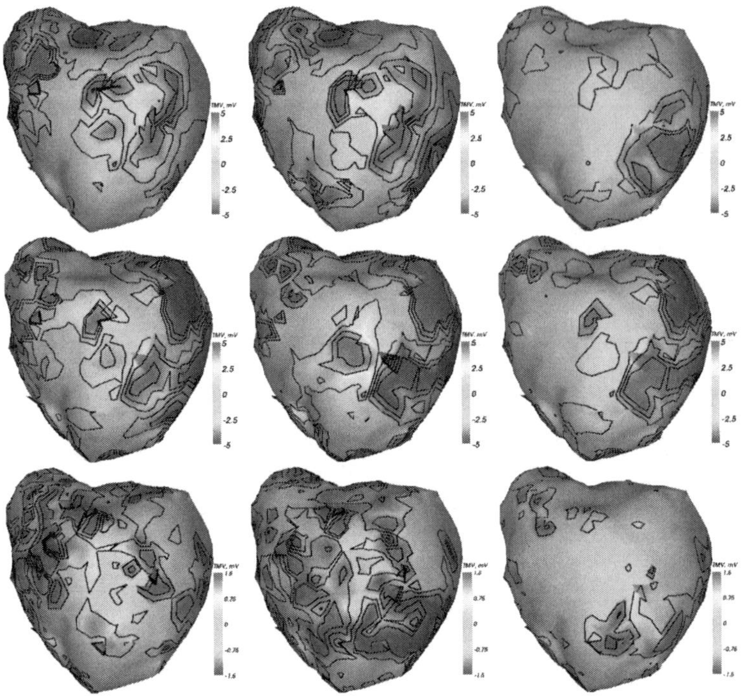

Figure 9.90: *Distributions of TMV reconstructed from the measured BSPMs using GM-Res (top), TG0 (middle) as well as TG2 (bottom) regularizations. Anterior view.*

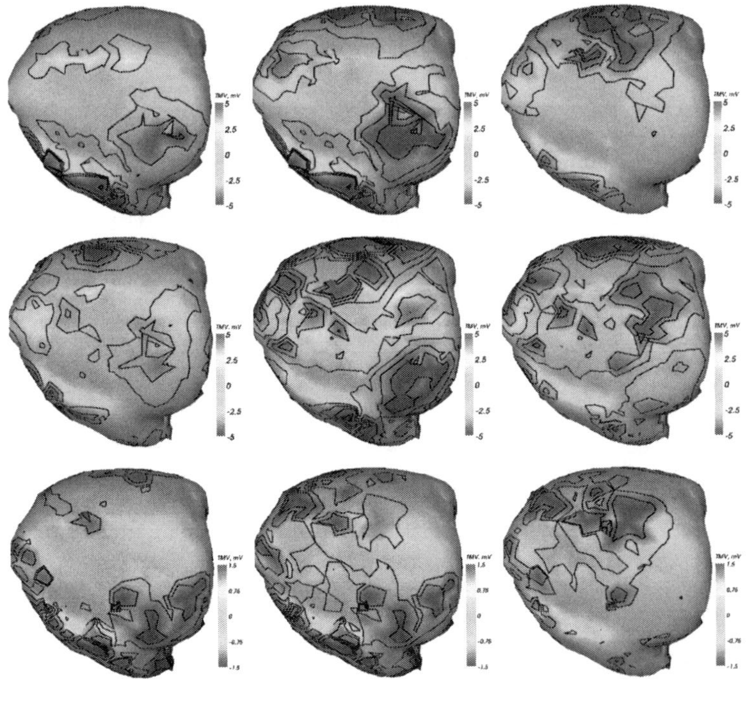

Figure 9.91: *Distributions of TMV reconstructed from the measured BSPMs using GM-Res (top), TG0 (middle) as well as TG2 (bottom) regularizations. Posterolateral view.*

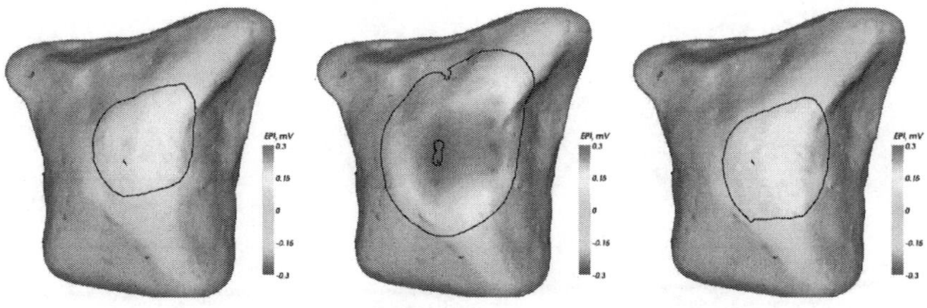

Figure 9.92: *Patient 5. BSPM during the T-wave.*

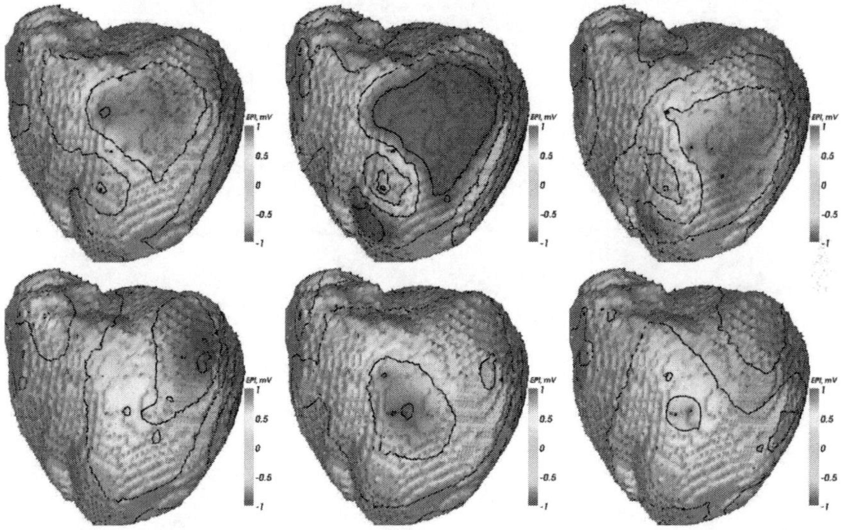

Figure 9.93: *Distributions of EP reconstructed from the measured BSPMs using GMRes regularization (top) as well as TG0 regularization (bottom). Anterior view.*

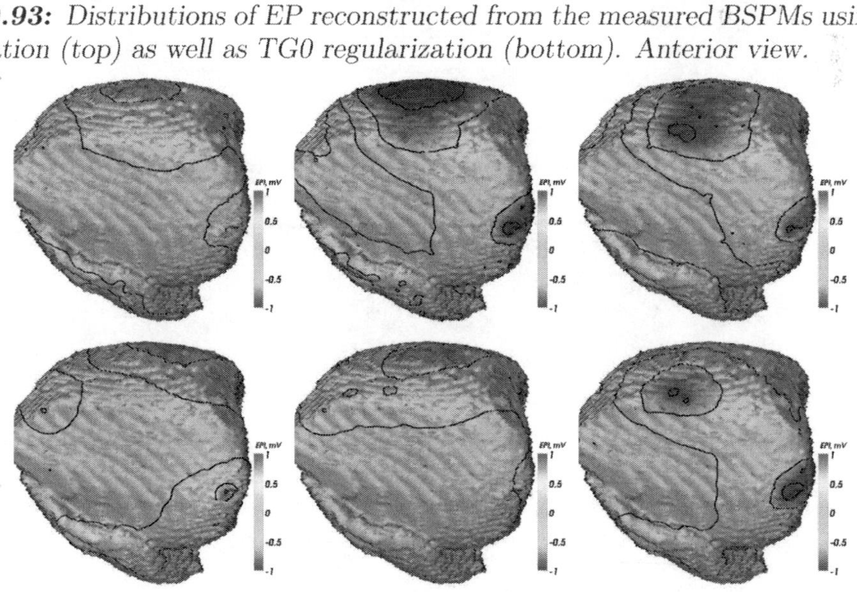

Figure 9.94: *Distributions of EP reconstructed from the measured BSPMs using GMRes regularization (top) as well as TG0 regularization (bottom). Posterolateral view.*

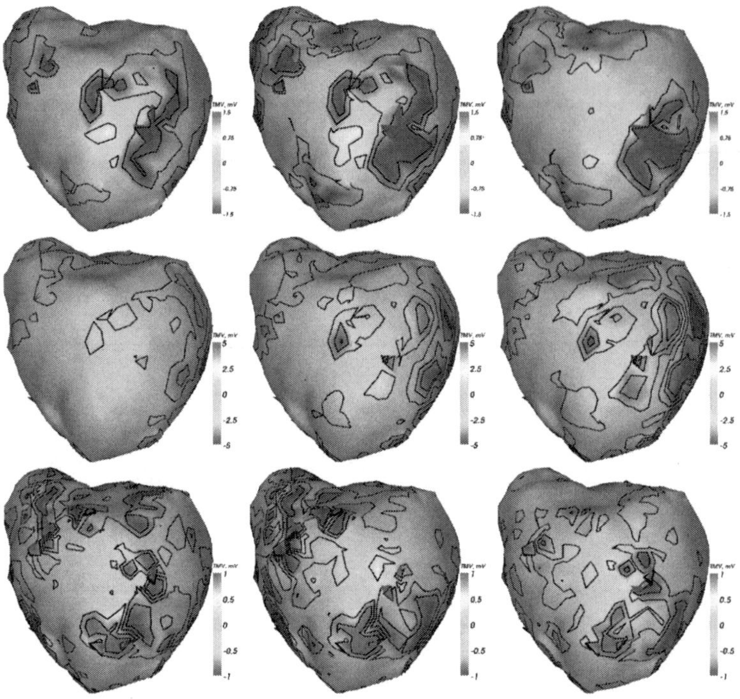

Figure 9.95: *Distributions of TMV reconstructed from the measured BSPMs using GM-Res (top), TG0 (middle) as well as TG2 (bottom) regularizations. Anterior view.*

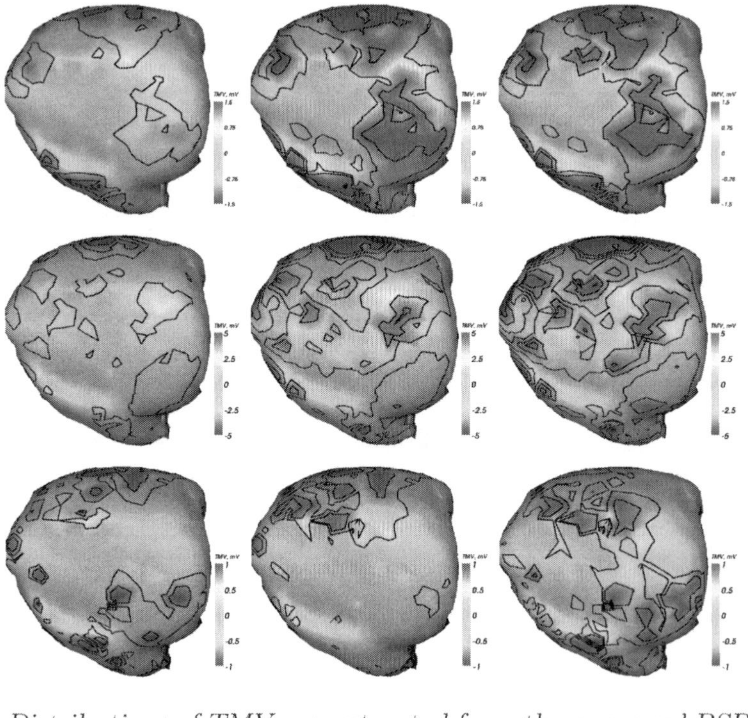

Figure 9.96: *Distributions of TMV reconstructed from the measured BSPMs using GM-Res (top), TG0 (middle) as well as TG2 (bottom) regularizations. Posterolateral view.*

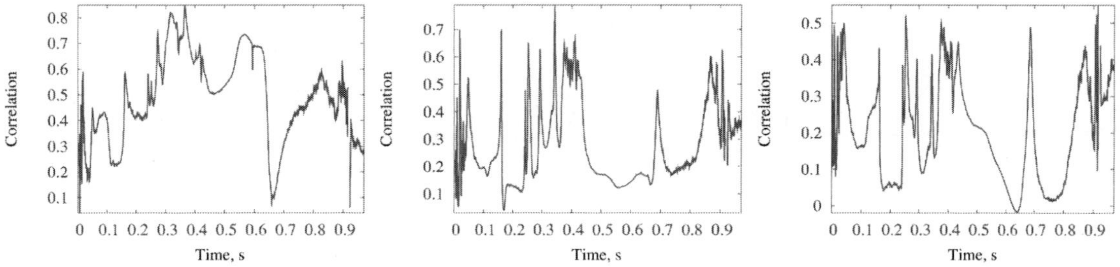

Figure 9.97: *Patient 5. Correlation between the reconstructed EP using GMRes vs. TG0 regularizations (left); between TMV distributions using GMRes vs. TG0 regularizations (middle); using TG2 vs. TG0 regularizations (right).*

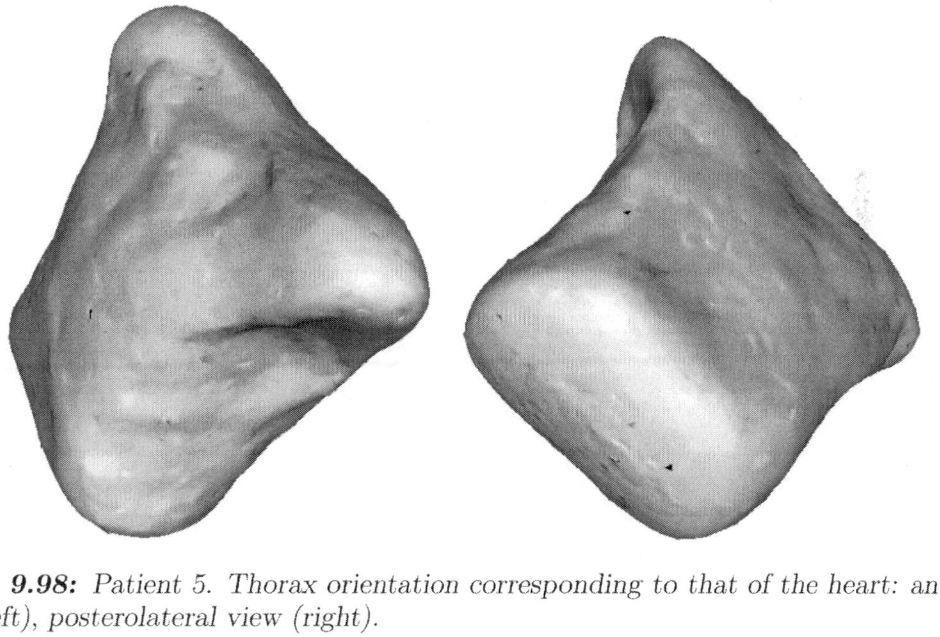

Figure 9.98: *Patient 5. Thorax orientation corresponding to that of the heart: anterior view (left), posterolateral view (right).*

Figure	Description	Color Range	Equipotential Lines
9.87	BSPM during QRS	-0.5..+0.5	-0.5, -0.3, ..., +0.5
9.88	EP during QRS ant.	-2..+2	-1.5, -0.5, +0.5, +1.5
9.89	EP during QRS post.	-2..+2	-1.5, -0.5, +0.5, +1.5
9.90	TMV during QRS ant.	-5..+5	-5, -3, -1, +1, +3, +5
	TMV during QRS ant. (TG2)	-1.5..+1.5	-1.5, -0.5, +0.5, +1.5
9.91	TMV during QRS post.	-5..+5	-5, -3, -1, +1, +3, +5
	TMV during QRS post. (TG2)	-1.5..+1.5	-1.5, -0.5, +0.5, +1.5
9.92	BSPM during T-wave	-0.3..+0.3	-0.3, -0.1, +0.1, +0.3
9.93	EP during T-wave ant.	-1..+1	-1, -0.6, ..., +1
9.94	EP during T-wave post.	-1..+1	-1, -0.6, ..., +1
9.95	TMV during T-wave ant. (GMRes)	-1.5..+1.5	-1.5, -0.5, +0.5, +1.5
	TMV during T-wave ant. (TG0)	-5..+5	-5, -3, ..., +5
	TMV during T-wave ant. (TG2)	-1..+1	-0.75, -0.25, +0.25, +0.75
9.96	TMV during T-wave post. (GMRes)	-1.5..+1.5	-1.5, -0.5, +0.5, +1.5
	TMV during T-wave post. (TG0)	-5..+5	-5, -3, ..., +5
	TMV during T-wave post. (TG2)	-1..+1	-0.75, -0.25, +0.25, +0.75

Table 9.3: *A short description, color range in mV, equipotential line values in mV for each of the figures representing the reconstruction results for patient 5. The reconstructed distributions of TMV are shown with different color scales for the sake of convenience.*

the case of TG0, that the propagation of excitation takes place from the right ventricle towards the left one.

The anterior surface of the left ventricle stays positive during the whole T-wave, the overall potential distribution during the repolarization is quite similar to that of the healthy subject (see figure 9.6). As this area has been excited later due to the left bundle branch block, it looks like the APD here is even smaller and/or the amplitude of excitation is lower. It can be explained by the physiological changes of the left ventricular myocardium caused by its dilation.

A small positive area is revealed by the GMRes technique on the anterior side of the heart, which might be a minor infarction area, but this observation is hardly supported by the TG0 case.

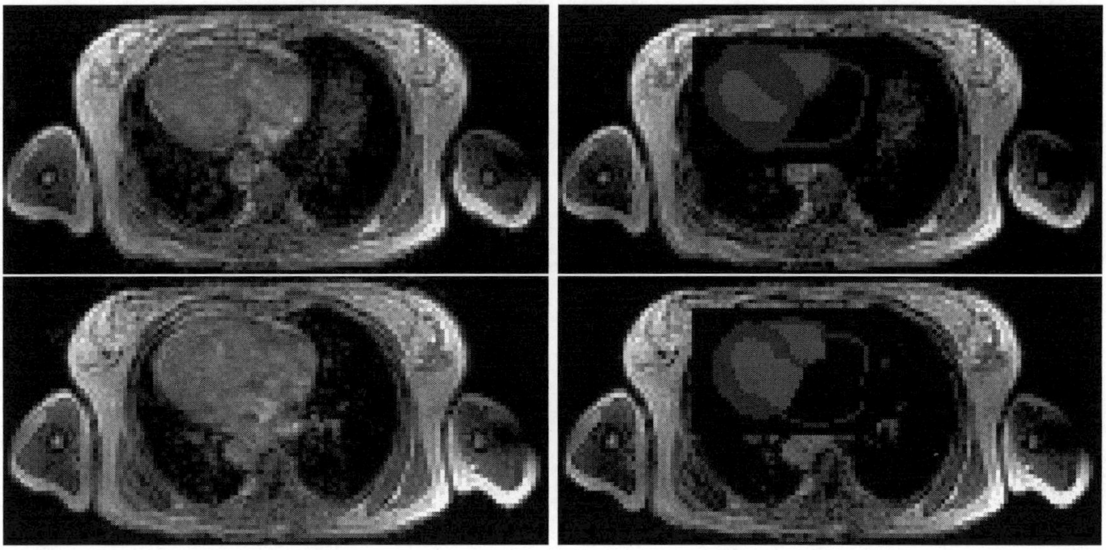

Figure 9.99: *Patient 6. Results of segmentation of the subject's heart (right) compared with the original SAX MRI data set (left). Top: near the ventricular base; bottom: near the apex.*

9.8 Patient 6

9.8.1 Description of the Patient and Segmentation Results

Patient 6, G.M., female, age 67, the location of infarction is unknown. The cardiac MRI data set has the resolution of $1.09 \times 1.09 \times 8.00\ mm^3$, contains 12 SAX-slices of 256×256 pixels. The MR-image of the thorax has the voxel size of $4 \times 4 \times 4\ mm^3$, includes 64 frontal slices of 128×128 pixels.

The heart has been segmented using the triangle meshes, the resulting anatomical model has the resolution of 1 mm. The atria are included schematically. The coordinate systems of thoracic and cardiac data sets do not correspond to each other, thus the relocation of the cardiac model had to be performed manually. Figure 9.99 demonstrates the cardiac model compared with the original MR-image of the thorax.

The tetrahedron mesh describing the patient's thorax contains 97,072 nodes and 594,469 tetrahedra. The average distance between nodes within myocardium is 2 mm. Lungs, heart, liver, spleen, kidneys, muscles and fat are segmented. The resulting thoracic model is compared with the original MRI data set in figure 9.100.

9.8.2 Measurement of BSPM

The 64-channel ECG was recorded with the sample rate of 2048 Hz during 200 s and processed by the averaging of multiple superimposed heart cycles. The resulting family of 64 ECG signals is shown in figure 9.101. Six dotted lines depict the time instants at which

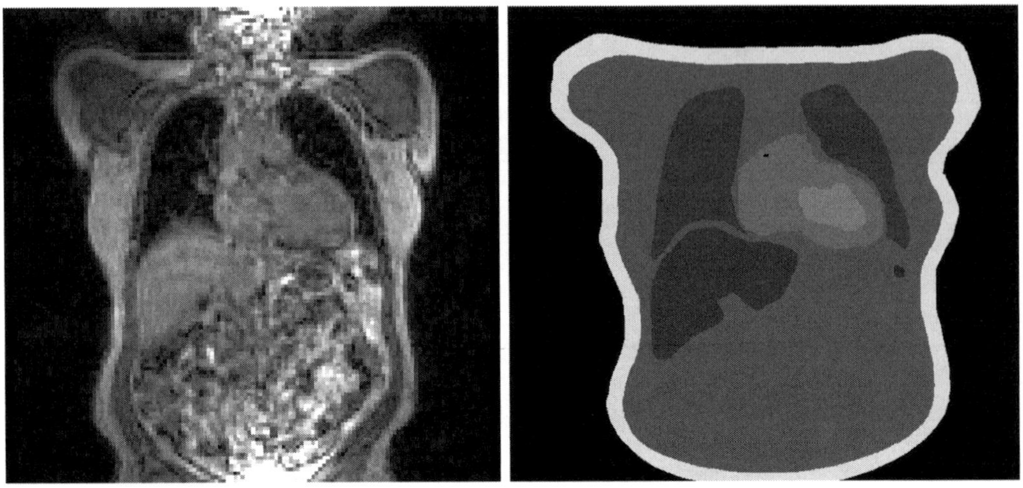

Figure 9.100: *Patient 6. Anatomical model of the subject's thorax (right) compared with the original data set (left).*

the interpolated BSPMs (figures 9.103 and 9.108) as well as the reconstructed distributions of EP and TMV are shown.

The standard leads built from this ECG are shown in figure 9.102. Due to anatomical reasons it was quite complicated to fix the electrodes in all the standard locations, therefore Wilson leads V1, V4 and V5 have not been measured.

9.8.3 Reconstruction Results

The distributions of endo- and epicardial potentials as well as transmembrane voltages reconstructed using different regularization methods are shown in figures 9.104-9.112. Table 9.4 contains short descriptions, color ranges and the values for isolines in these figures.

Figure	Description	Color Range	Equipotential Lines
9.103	BSPM during QRS	-0.3..+0.3	-0.3, -0.1, +0.1, +0.3
9.104	EP during QRS anterior	-1.5..+1.5	-1.5, -0.5, +0.5, +1.5
9.105	EP during QRS posterior	-1.5..+1.5	-1.5, -0.5, +0.5, +1.5
9.106	TMV during QRS anterior	-3..+3	-3, -1, +1, +3
9.107	TMV during QRS posterior	-3..+3	-3, -1, +1, +3
9.108	BSPM during T-wave	-0.05..+0.05	-0.05, -0.03, ..., +0.05
9.109	EP during T-wave anterior	-0.3..+0.3	-0.3, -0.1, +0.1, +0.3
9.110	EP during T-wave posterior	-0.3..+0.3	-0.3, -0.1, +0.1, +0.3
9.111	TMV during T-wave anterior	-1..+1	-1, -0.6, ..., +1
9.112	TMV during T-wave posterior	-1..+1	-1, -0.6, ..., +1

Table 9.4: *A short description, color range in mV, equipotential line values in mV for each of the figures representing the reconstruction results for patient 6.*

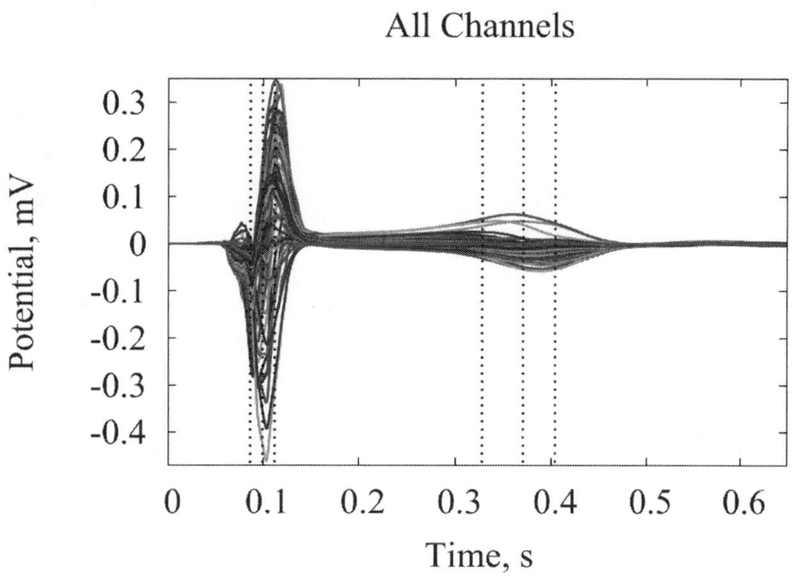

Figure 9.101: *Patient 6. ECG recorded with 64 measurement electrodes. Vertical dotted lines represent the time points at which the reconstruction was performed.*

The correlation between the distributions of equivalent cardiac sources obtained using different regularization techniques is shown in figure 9.113. The orientation of the patient's thorax corresponding to the anterior and posterolateral views of the heart is depicted in figure 9.114.

9.8.4 Conclusions

This is the most complicated case among the patients considered in the current work. First, the location of infarction has not been previously defined. Second, the locations of measurement electrodes had to be changed according to the anatomical features of the patient. Thus the number of electrodes in the immediate neighborhood of the heart had to be decreased, thus the spatial resolution of reconstructed sources was lower.

Still the correlation between the EP distributions reconstructed using TG0 vs. GMRes regularization methods is high for both QRS-complex and T-wave (0.9-0.95, see figure 9.113, left). These two methods also deliver quite similar results for the TMV distributions (same figure, center). Thus an assumption can be made that the quality of reconstruction is quite good.

Let us consider the depolarization phase. At the end of the QRS-complex a much later excitation of the lateral wall can be observed (figures 9.104-9.107). During the T-wave this area is the last to repolarize, a larger TMV (smaller EP) is keeping for a long time.

The posterior and posterolateral area is characterized by a lower TMV (higher EP)

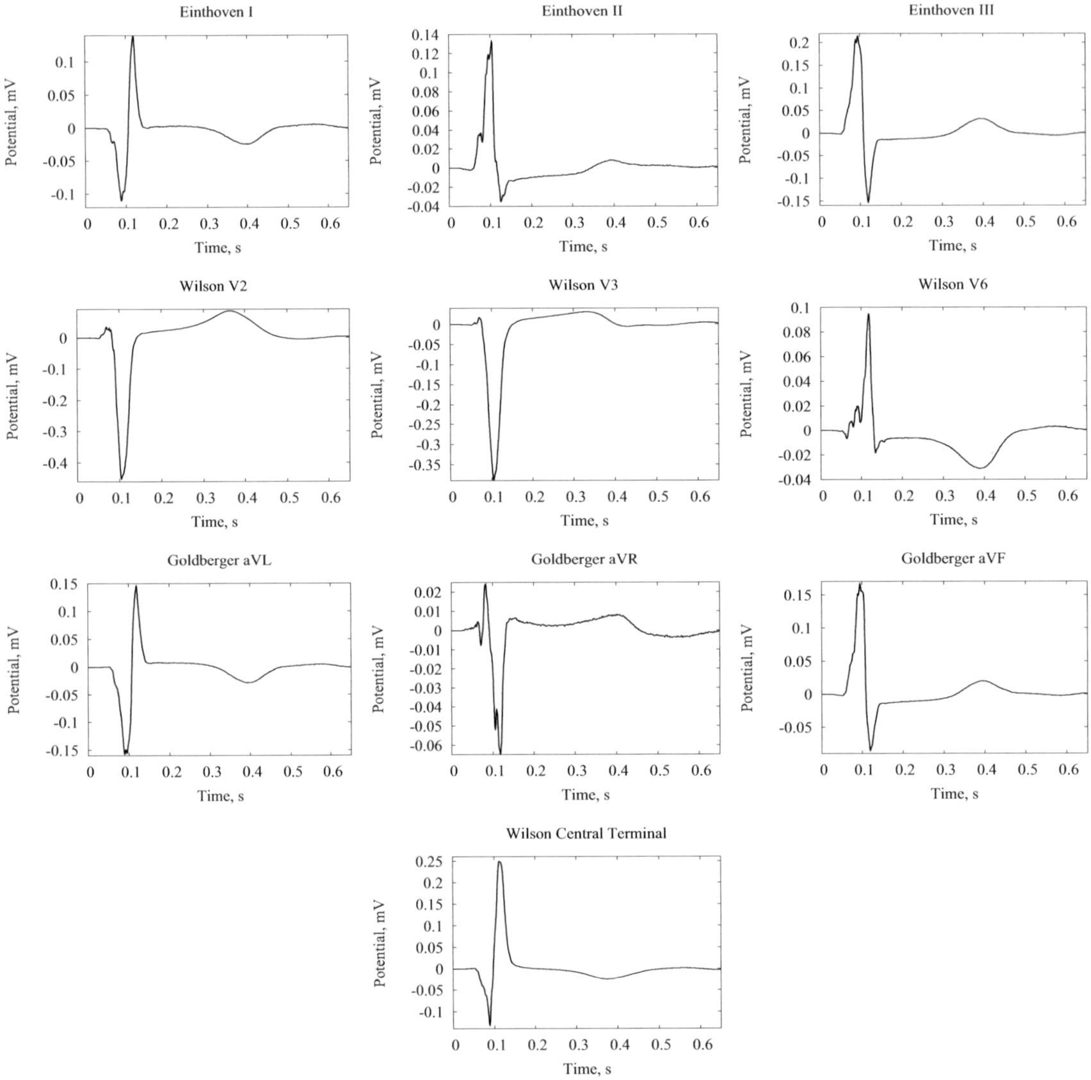

Figure 9.102: *Patient 6. Locations of the standard leads; 64-channel ECG; standard leads. There was no lead among the electrodes near enough to the standard electrode location V1, V4 and V5.*

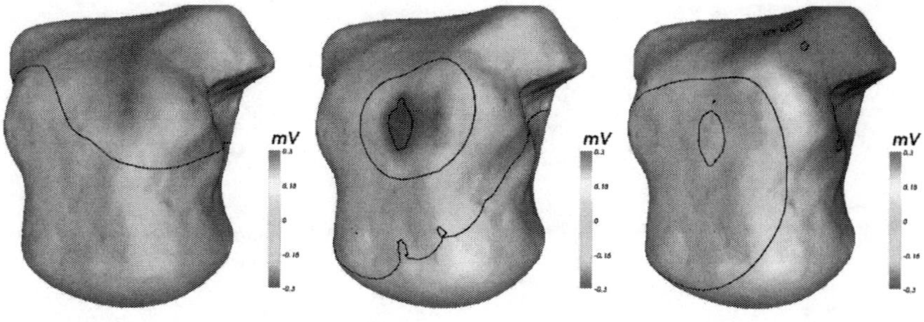

Figure 9.103: *Patient 6. Body surface potential maps (BSPM) during the QRS-complex. Time instants are marked in figure 9.101.*

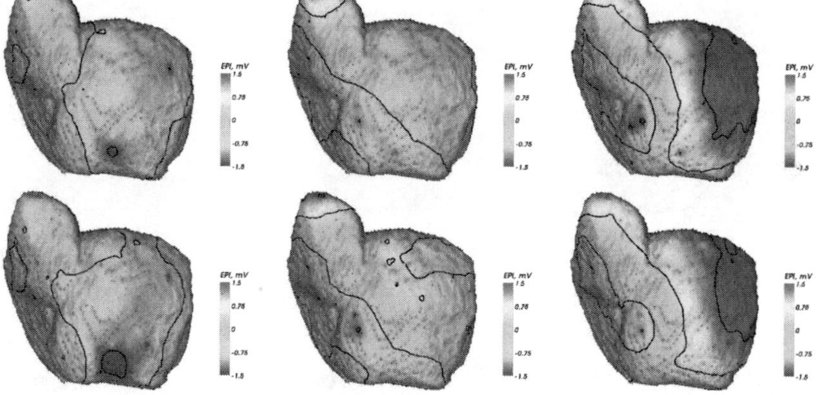

Figure 9.104: *Distributions of EP reconstructed from the measured BSPMs using GMRes (top) as well as TG0 (bottom) regularizations. Anterior view.*

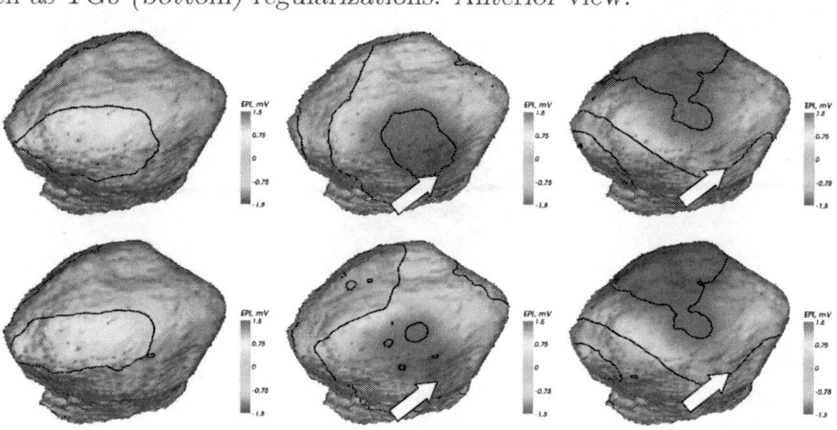

Figure 9.105: *Distributions of EP reconstructed from the measured BSPMs using GMRes (top) as well as TG0 (bottom) regularizations. Posterolateral view.*

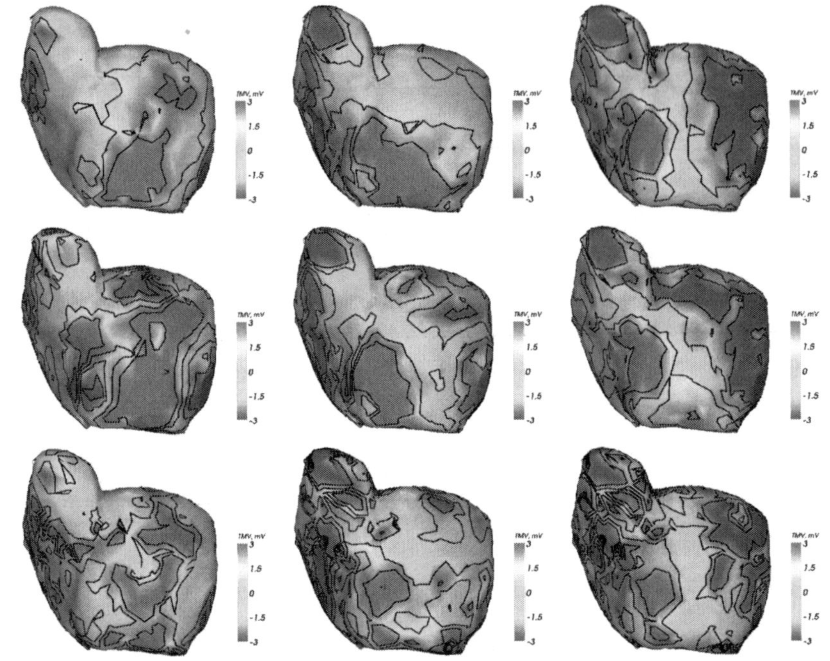

Figure 9.106: *Distributions of TMV reconstructed from the measured BSPMs using GMRes (top), TG0 (middle) as well as TG2 (bottom) regularizations. Anterior view.*

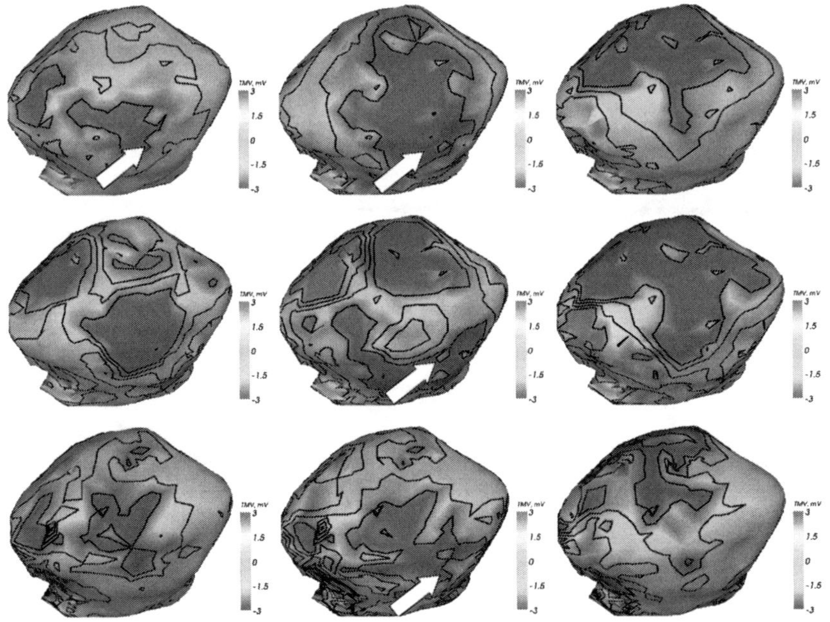

Figure 9.107: *Distributions of TMV reconstructed from the measured BSPMs using GMRes (top), TG0 (middle) as well as TG2 (bottom) regularizations. Posterolateral view.*

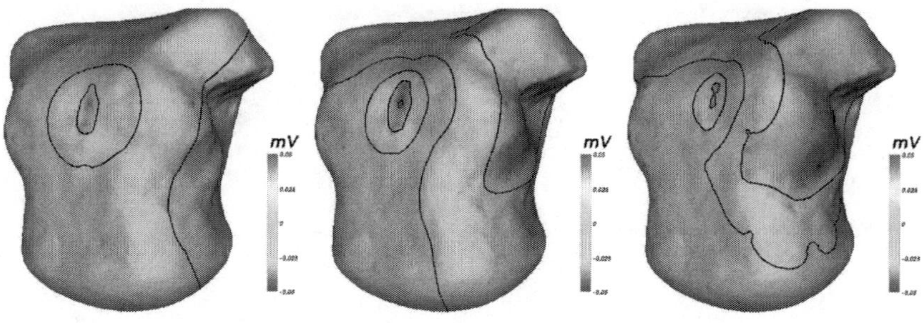

Figure 9.108: *Patient 6. BSPM during the T-wave. Time points* $t = 0.679,\ 0.718,\ 0.757$ *s are shown.*

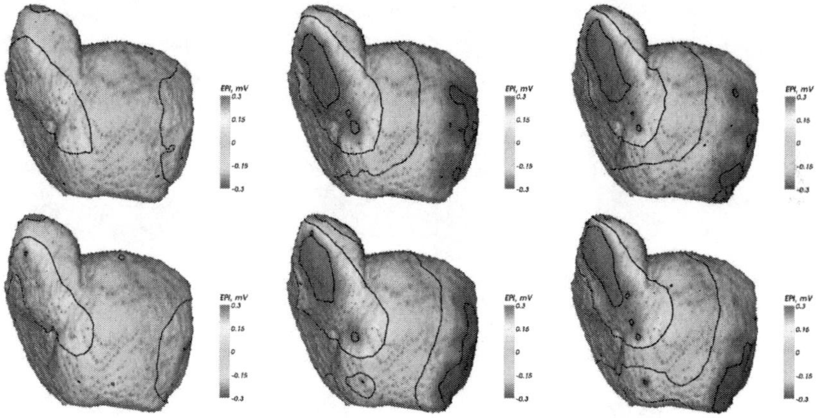

Figure 9.109: *Distributions of EP reconstructed from the measured BSPMs using GMRes regularization (top) as well as TG0 regularization (bottom). Anterior view.*

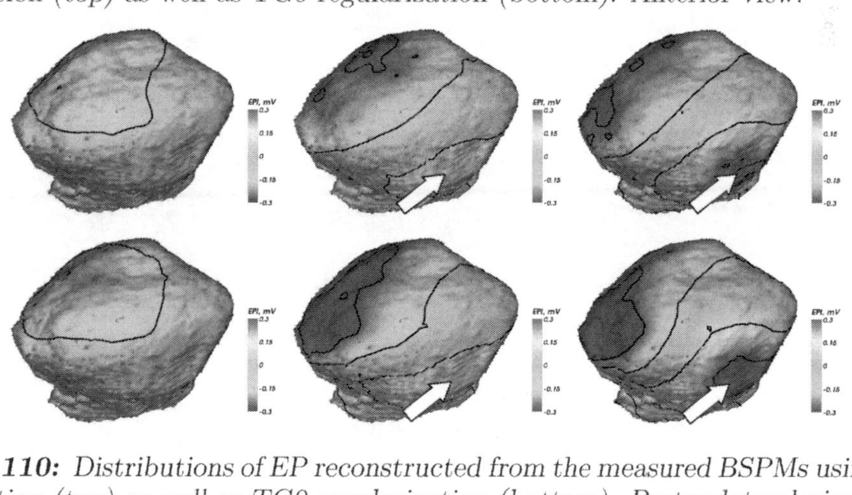

Figure 9.110: *Distributions of EP reconstructed from the measured BSPMs using GMRes regularization (top) as well as TG0 regularization (bottom). Posterolateral view.*

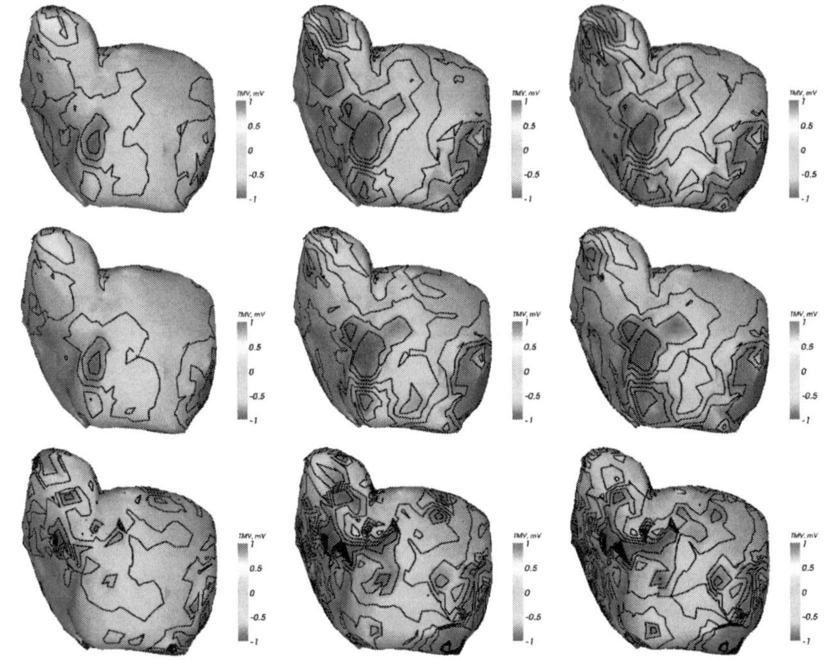

Figure 9.111: *Distributions of TMV reconstructed from the measured BSPMs using GMRes (top), TG0 (middle) as well as TG2 (bottom) regularizations. Anterior view.*

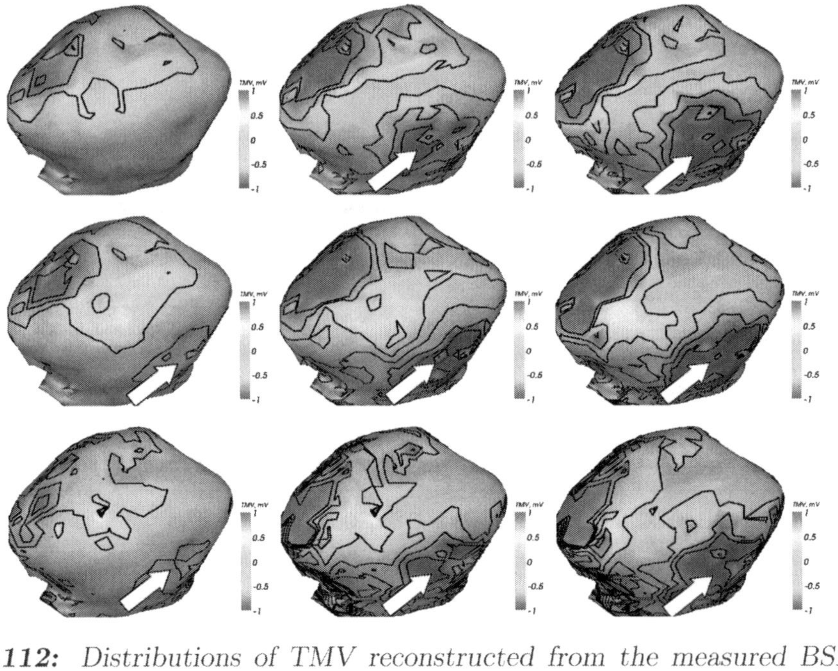

Figure 9.112: *Distributions of TMV reconstructed from the measured BSPMs using GMRes (top), TG0 (middle) as well as TG2 (bottom) regularizations. Posterolateral view.*

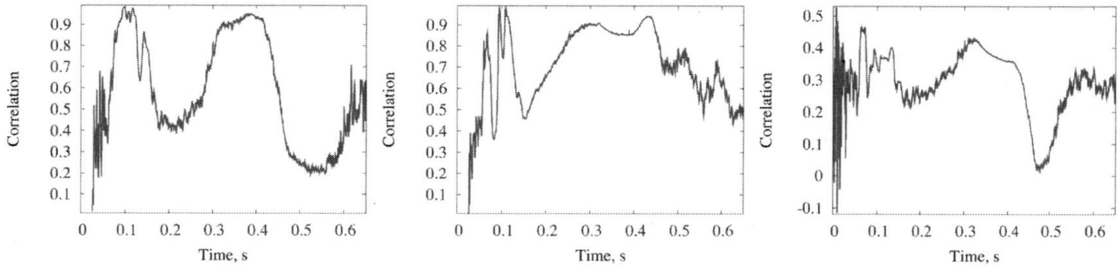

Figure 9.113: *Patient 6. Correlation between the reconstructed EP using GMRes vs. TG0 regularizations (left); between TMV distributions using GMRes vs. TG0 regularizations (middle); using TG2 vs. TG0 regularizations (right).*

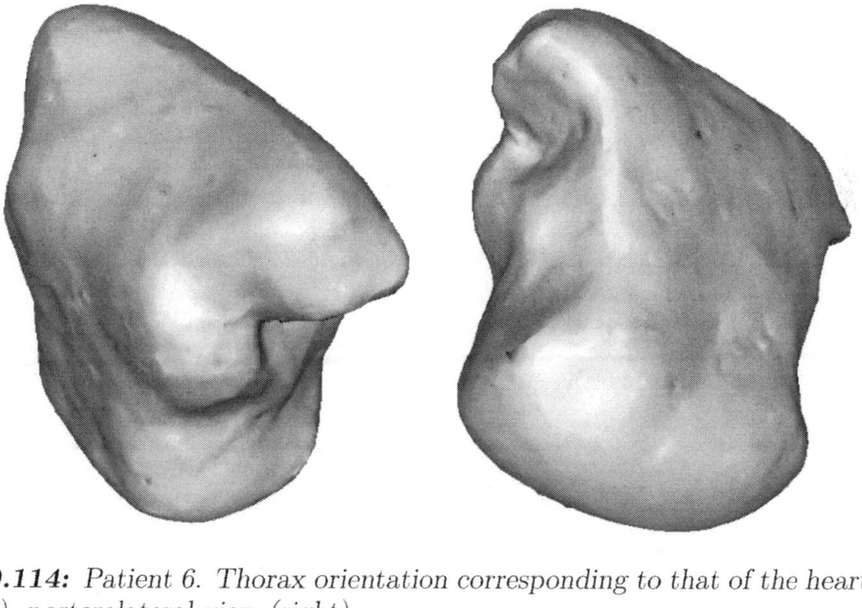

Figure 9.114: *Patient 6. Thorax orientation corresponding to that of the heart: anterior view (left), posterolateral view (right).*

throughout the cardiac cycle. Therefore the following assumption can be made. The infarction scar is located in the posterolateral area of the heart. The infarction is transmural, and the left posterior fascicle is at least partially blocked. This leads to a later excitation (and relaxation) of the lateral wall.

9.9 Patient 7

9.9.1 Description of the Patient and Segmentation Results

Patient 7, A.Z., male, age 48, suffers from anterior infarction. The cardiac MRI data set had the resolution of $0.98 \times 0.98 \times 6.00\ mm^3$ and contained 24 SAX-images of 256×256 pixels. The resolution of the thoracic data set was $4 \times 4 \times 4\ mm^3$, with 64 frontal snapshots of 128×128 pixels.

The segmentation of these data sets was performed using deformable triangle meshes. The atria were not included into the cardiac MRI data set, thus they were segmented schematically. The resulting anatomical model of patient's heart has the isotropic resolution of 1 mm. This model is compared with the original MRI data set in figure 9.115.

The finite element mesh representing the anatomy of the thorax contains 95,933 nodes and 585,664 tetrahedra, the distance between neighboring nodes within the ventricular myocardium is 2 mm. Heart, lungs, liver, spleen, kidneys, muscles and fat have been segmented. The resulting structure of the volume conductor is compared with the original MR-image in figure 9.116.

9.9.2 Measurement of BSPM

The BSPM was recorded using the same 64-electrode BioSemi system. Several sequences 200 s long with the sample rate of 2048 Hz were made. In each channel the single ECG cycles were cut out, superimposed and averaged. Resulting 64-channel ECG is shown in figure 9.117. Six dotted lines denote the time instants at which the BSPMs as well as the reconstruction results are shown.

The standard ECG leads extracted from the measured data set is shown in figure 9.118. Wilson lead V4 has not been built as there has been no electrode located near it.

The BSPMs interpolated on the whole surface of the thorax are shown in figures 9.119 (QRS-complex) and 9.124 (T-wave).

9.9.3 Reconstruction Results

The reconstructed distributions of EP and TMV are shown in figures 9.120-9.128. Short descriptions of these figures, chosen color ranges and the values for isolines are listed in table 9.5.

Figure 9.129 depicts the correlation between the distributions of epicardial potentials (left) or transmembrane voltages (middle, right) obtained using different regularization methods. The distributions of EP show a very good correlation during the whole heart cycle (0.8-0.9). The correlation curve for TMV (TG0 vs. GMRes regularization) demonstrates two peaks for the QRS-complex and T-wave of about 0.8, the rest of the time the correlation changes quite chaotically. The correlation between the TMV distributions obtained using TG0 and TG2 regularization methods is quite constant with the value of about 0.45.

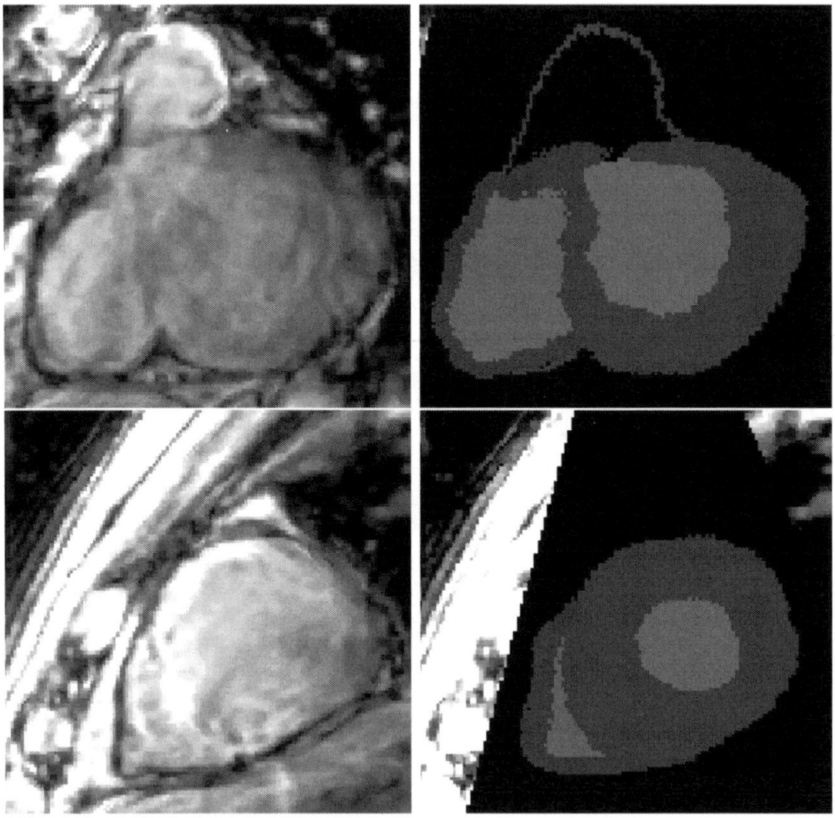

Figure 9.115: *Patient 7. Results of segmentation of the subject's heart (right) compared with the original SAX MRI data set (left). Top: near the ventricular base; bottom: near the apex.*

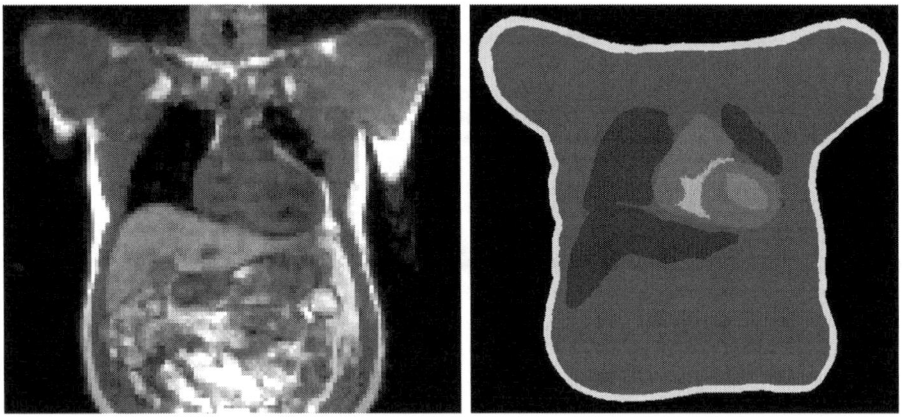

Figure 9.116: *Patient 7. Anatomical model of the subject's thorax (right) compared with the original data set (left).*

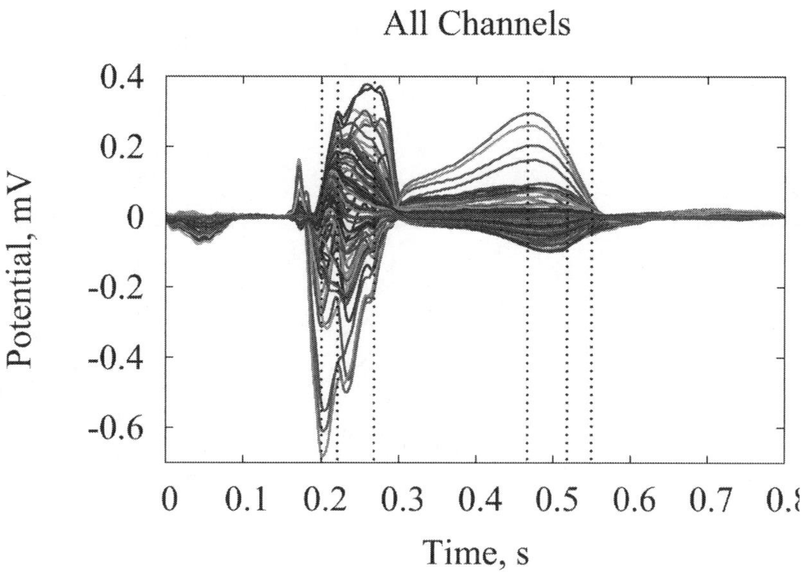

Figure 9.117: *Patient 7. ECG recorded with 64 measurement electrodes. Vertical dotted lines represent the time points at which the reconstruction was performed.*

Figure	Description	Color Range	Equipotential Lines
9.119	BSPM during QRS	-0.3..+0.3	-0.3, -0.1, +0.1, +0.3
9.120	EP during QRS anterior	-1..+1	-1, -0.6, ..., +1
9.121	EP during QRS posterior	-1..+1	-1, -0.6, ..., +1
9.122	TMV during QRS ant. (GMRes)	-3..+3	-3, -1, +1, +3
	TMV during QRS ant. (TG0, TG2)	-6..+6	-6, -2, +2, +6
9.123	TMV during QRS post. (GMRes)	-3..+3	-3, -1, +1, +3
	TMV during QRS post. (TG0, TG2)	-6..+6	-6, -2, +2, +6
9.124	BSPM during T-wave	-0.1..+0.1	-0.1, -0.06, ..., +0.1
9.125	EP during T-wave anterior	-0.5..+0.5	-0.5, -0.3, ..., +0.5
9.126	EP during T-wave posterior	-0.5..+0.5	-0.5, -0.3, ..., +0.5
9.127	TMV during T-wave ant. (GMRes)	-1.5..+1.5	-1.5, -0.5, +0.5, +1.5
	TMV during T-wave ant. (TG0, TG2)	-3..+3	-3, -1, +1, +3
9.128	TMV during T-wave post. (GMRes)	-1.5..+1.5	-1.5, -0.5, +0.5, +1.5
	TMV during T-wave post. (TG0, TG2)	-3..+3	-3, -1, +1, +3

Table 9.5: *Short descriptions, color ranges in mV, equipotential line values in mV for each of the figures representing the reconstruction results for patient 7.*

The orientation of the thorax corresponding to that of the heart for anterior and posterolateral views is shown in figure 9.130.

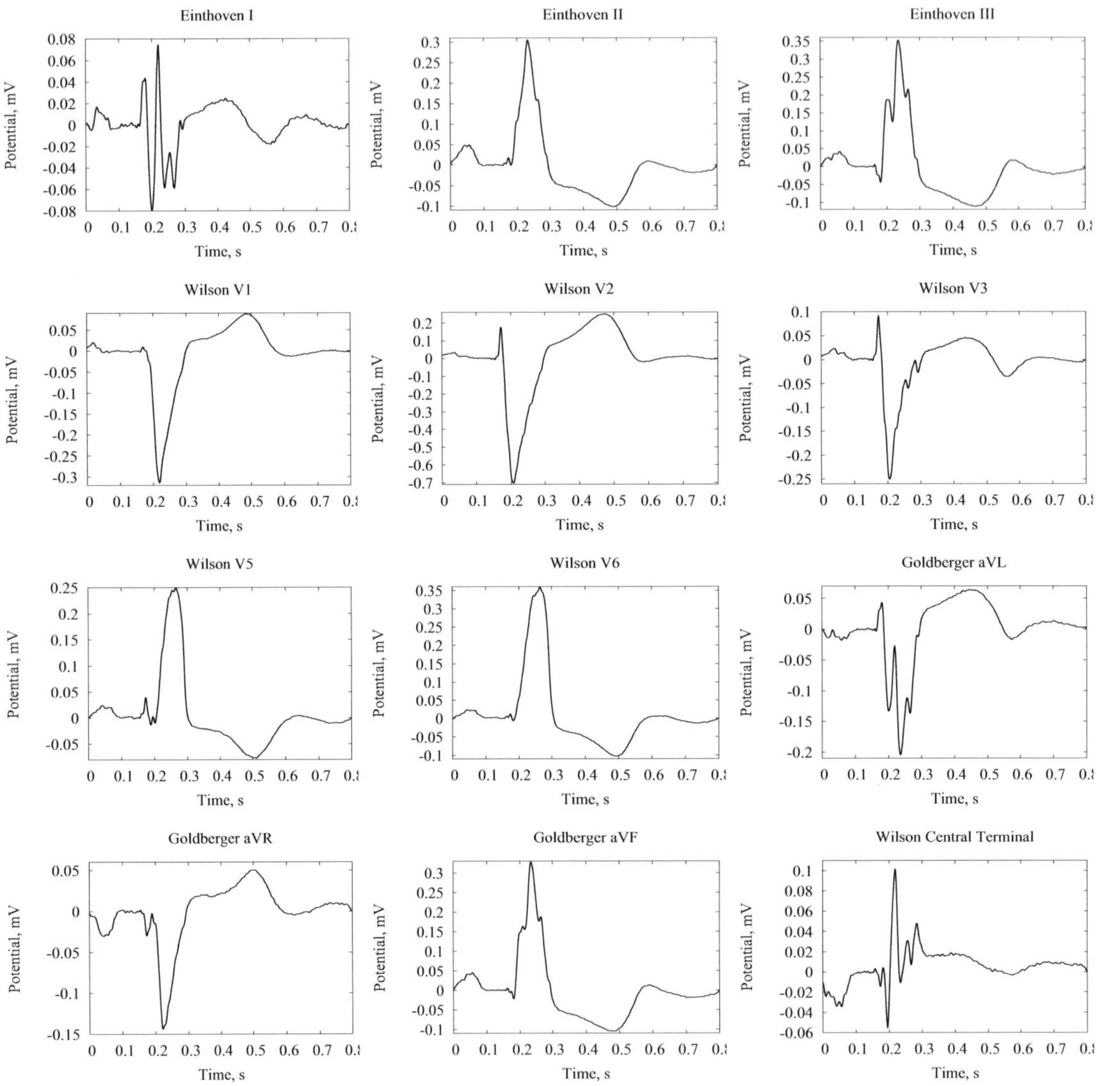

Figure 9.118: *Patient 7. Locations of the standard leads; 64-channel ECG; standard leads. There was no lead among the electrodes near enough to the standard electrode location V4.*

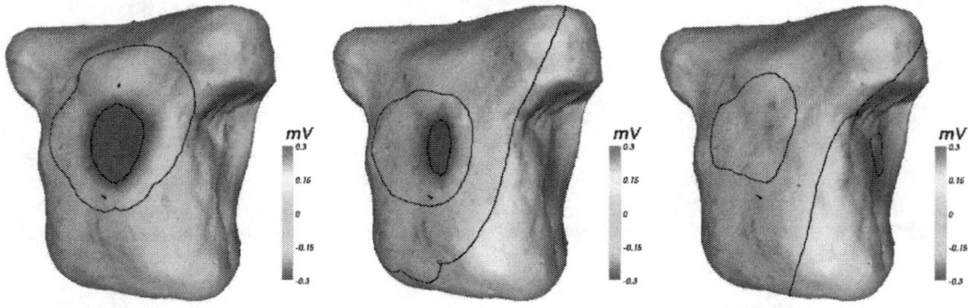

Figure 9.119: *Patient 7. Body surface potential maps (BSPM) during the QRS-complex. Time instants are marked in figure 9.117.*

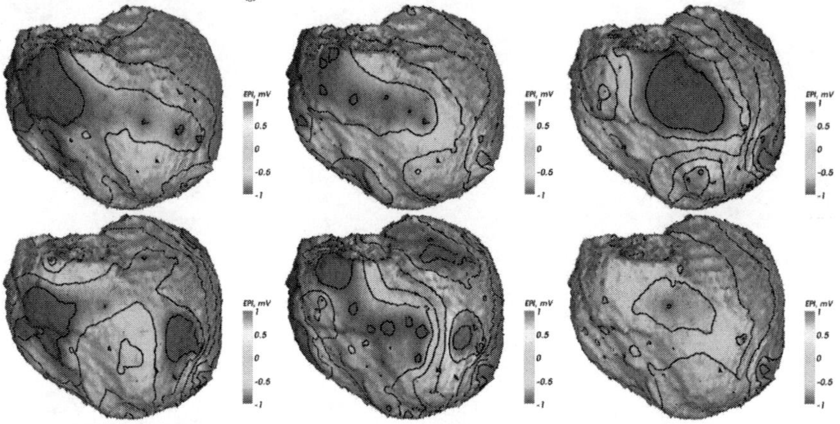

Figure 9.120: *Distributions of EP reconstructed from the measured BSPMs using GMRes (top) as well as TG0 (bottom) regularizations. Anterior view.*

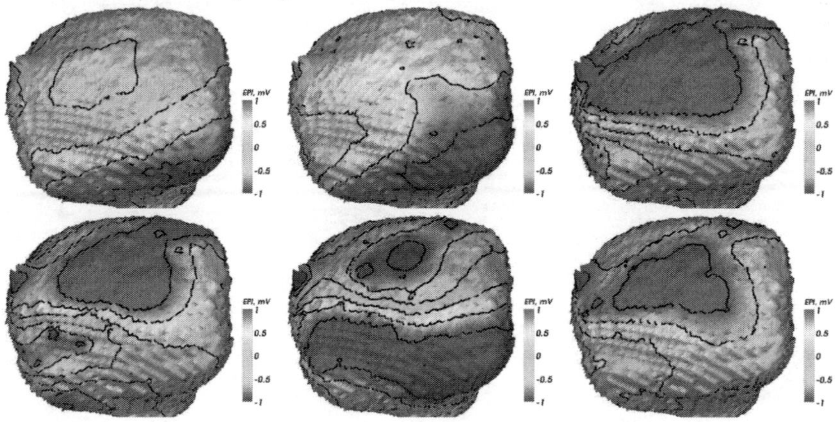

Figure 9.121: *Distributions of EP reconstructed from the measured BSPMs using GMRes (top) as well as TG0 (bottom) regularizations. Posterolateral view.*

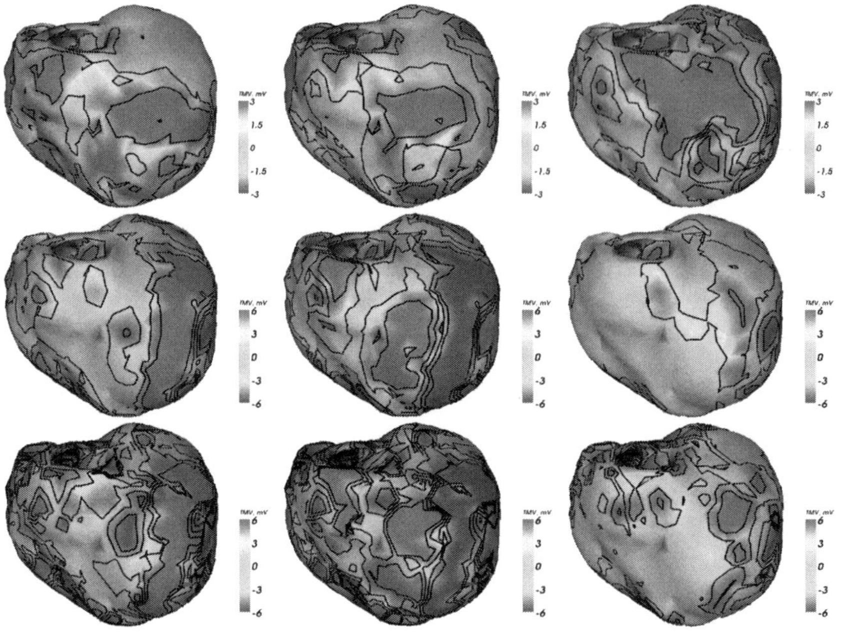

Figure 9.122: *Distributions of TMV reconstructed from the measured BSPMs using GMRes (top), TG0 (middle) as well as TG2 (bottom) regularizations. Anterior view.*

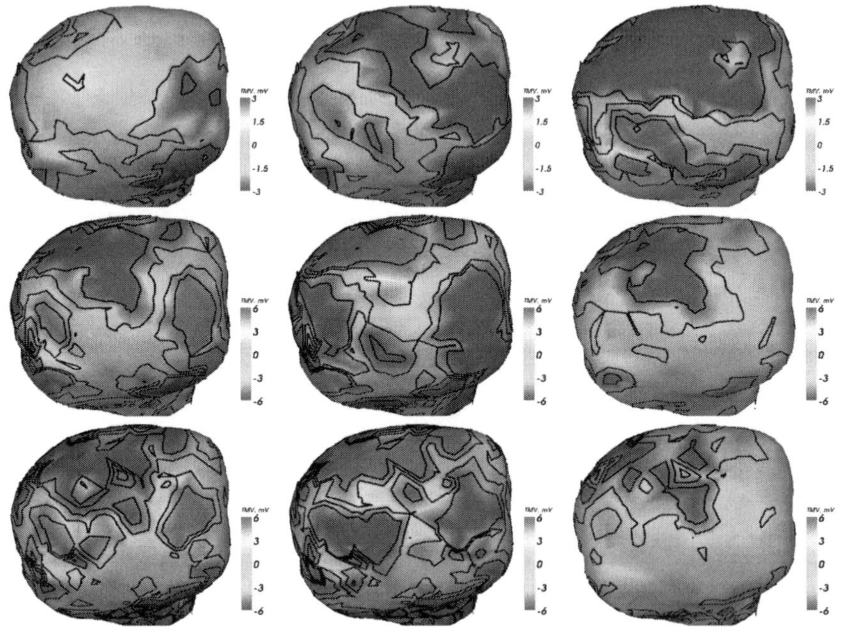

Figure 9.123: *Distributions of TMV reconstructed from the measured BSPMs using GMRes (top), TG0 (middle) as well as TG2 (bottom) regularizations. Posterolateral view.*

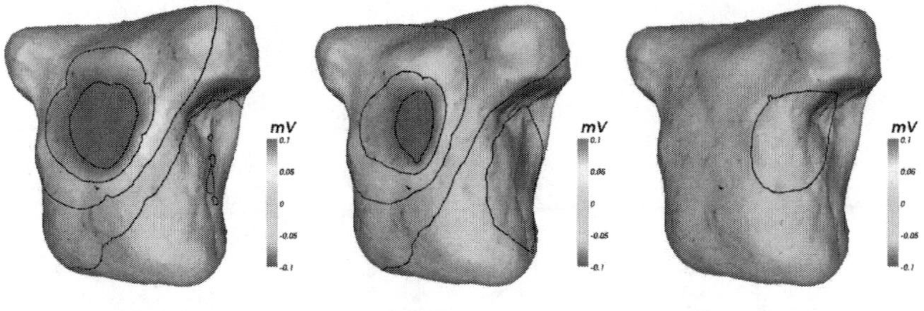

Figure 9.124: *Patient 7. BSPM during the T-wave.*

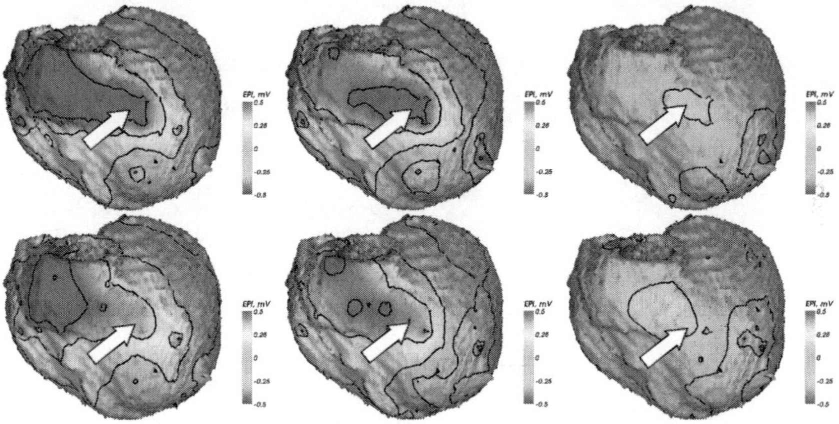

Figure 9.125: *Distributions of EP reconstructed from the measured BSPMs using GMRes regularization (top) as well as TG0 regularization (bottom). Anterior view.*

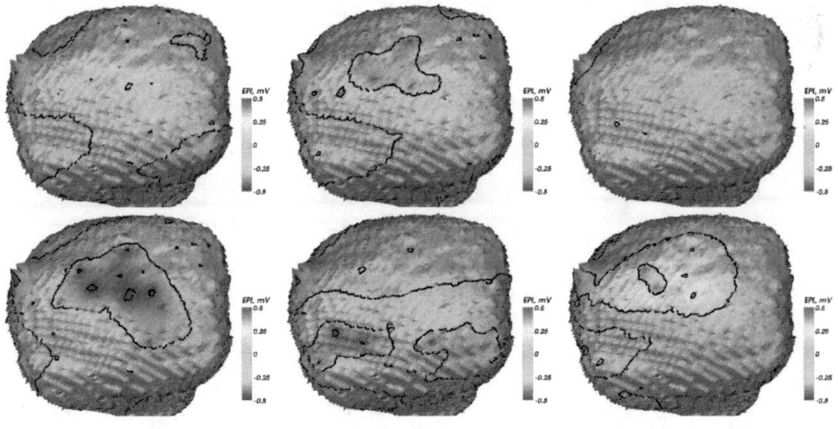

Figure 9.126: *Distributions of EP reconstructed from the measured BSPMs using GMRes regularization (top) as well as TG0 regularization (bottom). Posterolateral view.*

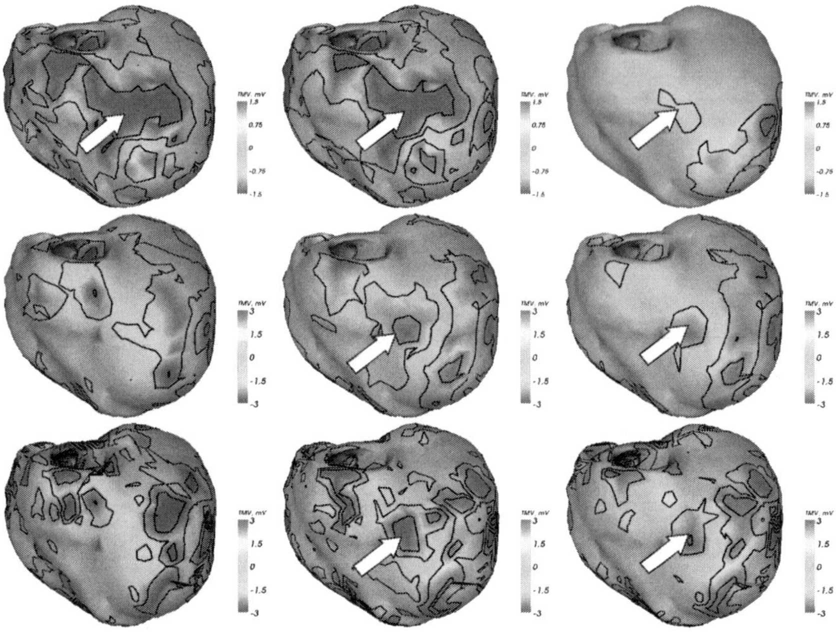

Figure 9.127: *Distributions of TMV reconstructed from the measured BSPMs using GMRes (top), TG0 (middle) as well as TG2 (bottom) regularizations. Anterior view.*

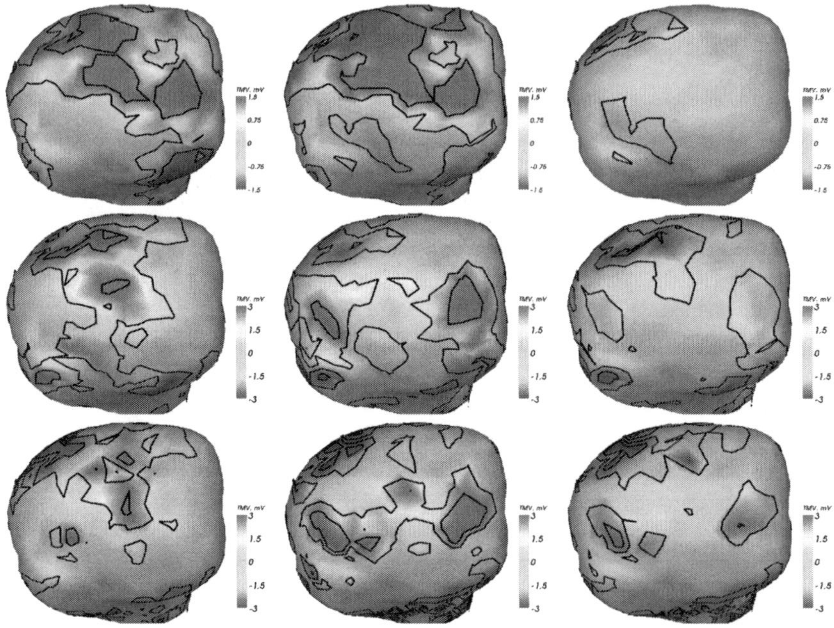

Figure 9.128: *Distributions of TMV reconstructed from the measured BSPMs using GMRes (top), TG0 (middle) as well as TG2 (bottom) regularizations. Posterolateral view.*

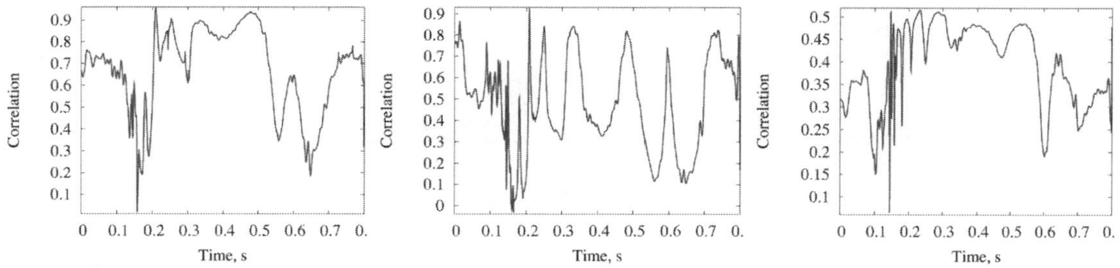

Figure 9.129: *Patient 7. Correlation between the reconstructed EP using GMRes vs. TG0 regularizations (left); between TMV distributions using GMRes vs. TG0 regularizations (middle); using TG2 vs. TG0 regularizations (right).*

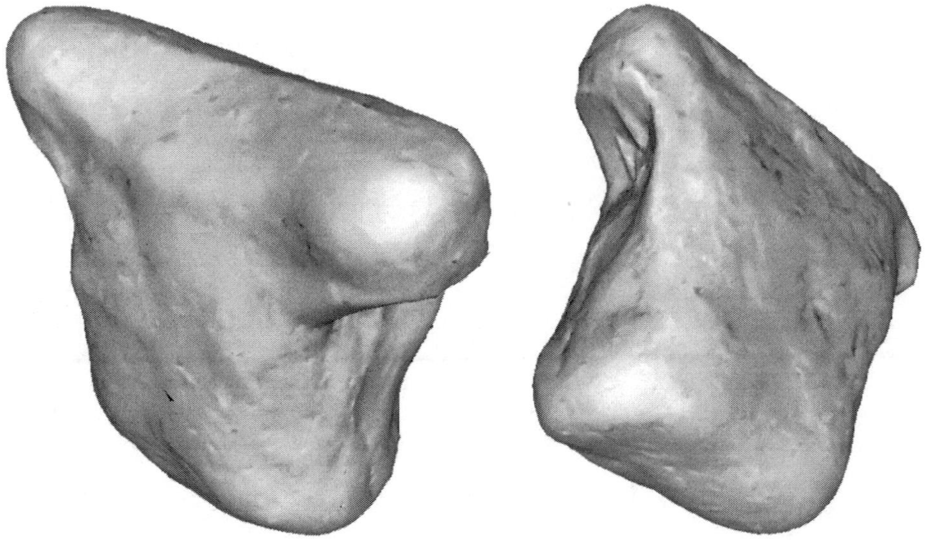

Figure 9.130: *Patient 7. Thorax orientation corresponding to that of the heart: anterior view (left), posterolateral view (right).*

9.9.4 Conclusions

The correlation between the distributions of epicardial potentials obtained using TG0 vs. GMRes regularization methods is quite high during the whole heart cycle (0.8-0.9, see figure 9.129, left), whereas for the TMV case the correlation is somewhat lower (0.5-0.8, figure 9.129, center and right).

During the T-wave an area with a smaller TMV (higher EP) can be observed on the anterior wall (figures 9.125, 9.127). The difference is evident all through the ST-interval. This area is shown to be excited only during the QRS-complex (9.120, 9.122), where the correct reconstruction of cardiac sources is complicated. Thus a conclusion can be made that the anterior infarction has been detected.

The de- and repolarization of the lateral wall takes place with a quite large delay. This might happen due to the left bundle branch block caused by the anterior infarction. Also the comparison of the leads V4-V6 of patient 7 are very similar to those of patient 5 with the left bundle branch block.

Chapter 10

Discussion and Outlook

Several methods of noninvasive reconstruction of cardiac activity have been presented in the current work. They can be subdivided primarily into three different strategies:

1. Optimization-based approach: an electrophysiological cardiac model is created, its parameters are varied until the simulated ECG gets similar to the measured one.
2. Solution of the inverse problem of electrocardiography: the matrix equation describing the (linear) relationship between the distribution of cardiac sources and BSPM is solved with minimal *a priori* information involved.
3. The results of modeling are used as *a priori* statistical information in order to stabilize the solution of the inverse problem.

Each of these approaches has its advantages and disadvantages. The features of each approach and the future work are described in the following sections.

10.1 Optimization-Based Methods

The optimization-based approach is quite time-consuming: up to several thousand simulations are to be made in order to obtain a satisfactory correspondence between the model and reality. Each step takes up to half an hour of computation time, thus the whole computation can take several weeks.

Another feature of this approach is a high vulnerability to modeling errors. It is important to create a nearly perfect model of, say, myocardial infarction, left bundle branch block or distribution of action potential duration, flexible enough but characterized by a relatively small number of parameters, otherwise the time needed for optimization increases rapidly.

Still the solution of this problem delivers the physician a fully functioning model of the cardiac activity specific for the patient under consideration. Based on this model, important conclusions can be made about the future development of the disease, for example an estimation of the stability of the heart function can be made.

The cellular automaton based approach employed in the current work provides enough flexibility for such modeling, whereas the computation time is relatively low, compared to the methods based on bidomain models.

The following improvements are to be introduced into the method in the course of future work. First, a more flexible way to define the distribution of action potential duration is to be introduced. Second, the models of various heart diseases must be implemented, in cooperation with clinical cardiologists. This work is already being done within the scope of several projects. Particularly, intracardiac catheter measurements are to be performed. These measurements must improve our knowledge about the cardiac activity, especially in different pathological cases. This would allow to strongly enhance the presented models.

10.2 Inverse Problem of Electrocardiography

The solution of the inverse problem is an alternative way to obtain information about the cardiac activity noninvasively. It requires the development of an anatomical model of the patient's thorax, correct positioning of measurement electrodes on its surface and relatively accurate measurements of multichannel ECG. The whole time needed to solve the inverse problem of electrocardiography for a specific patient can be estimated at one till two workdays of a single researcher.

Two tasks are most time-consuming in the course of reconstruction: the segmentation of the 3D data set describing the anatomy of the patient and the computation of the transfer matrix which is to be inverted (see chapter 5). Recent progress in methods of automatic segmentation (see, e.g., [45, 49, 168]) can significantly reduce the time needed to create an anatomical model. The computation of the transfer matrix is easily scalable for any number of CPUs, thus the problem can be technically solved as well.

The solution of the inverse problem delivers the distributions of cardiac sources at each time instant. The usefulness of this information has been demonstrated in chapter 9, where patients with various cardiac diseases were considered. Thus the method is able to increase the precision of medical diagnostics.

The future research will be performed in the following directions. First, intracardiac catheter measurements will be done. These data along with the measurement of BSPM must provide a much better spatial resolution for the solution of the inverse problem. Thus an important information will be obtained for the modeling of various heart diseases, as it was described in the previous section.

Second, new methods must be implemented to reconstruct the cardiac sources. They include the computation of activation times for the cardiac surface and eventually for the whole volume of myocardium, like it is done in [119, 169]. Another interesting approach is the temporal regularization based on the assumption of monotonically nondecreasing (during depolarization) or nonincreasing (for the repolarization phase) transmembrane voltage in each point of the myocardium ([117], see section 5.3). Both of these methods pose a much more strict bias on the solution of the inverse problem, thus a better stabilization is achieved.

Third, a standardization of cardiac sources locations has to be done. Only visual comparison between the distributions of heart surface potentials or transmembrane voltages for different cardiac geometries can currently be performed, like it has been shown in chapter 9. Of course, an exact comparison cannot be performed in this way. Instead, a universal mesh describing the myocardial surface (triangular) or volume (tetrahedral) has to be constructed, which should be further deformed in order to match the cardiac geometry of any patient. Thus the automatic comparison between different distributions of cardiac sources can be performed.

10.3 MAP-Regularization

The *maximum a posteriori* regularization is a particular method of solution of the inverse problem. An important aspect consists in the employment of *a priori* estimation of the solution (see section 5.3). The development of the statistical basis in order to build the estimator can take several days, whereas this task can easily be parallelized for any reasonable number of processing units. Not only can the runs of simulation with different parameters be performed independently on different workstations, each simulation is actually also able to employ several processors.

If the real cardiac activity of the patient is close enough to some estimations belonging to the statistical basis, the quality of reconstruction increases dramatically compared to the common regularization methods (Tikhonov, GMRes). Such a comparison has been performed within the scope of this work, e.g., in [134, 138, 140].

The condition that the real distribution of cardiac sources belongs to the statistical basis of estimations is quite important. Still even a simple *a priori* assumption about the characteristics of the cardiac disease allows a physician to reduce the size of the statistical basis significantly. This leads to a stronger biasing and thus to a better stabilization of the problem.

Thus although the MAP-regularization method takes more time for the solution of the inverse problem compared to Tikhonov or GMRes, the time consumption is much lower than that for the optimization-based method. Afterwards the resulting information (say, the configuration of infarction scar) can be used in modeling.

On the other hand, this method delivers much more reliable information than the common regularization methods. Thus in spite of a larger time consumption it might be very useful in everyday clinical practice.

Bibliography

[1] C. L. Schlauf, D. F. Moffet, and S. B. Moffet, *Medizinische Physiologie.* Walter de Gruyter, Berlin, 1997.

[2] A. A. Young, L. J. LeGrice, M. A. Young, and B. H. Smaill, "Extended confocal microscopy of myocardial laminae and collagen network," *J. Microscopy*, vol. 192, pp. 139–150, Nov. 1998.

[3] D. D. Streeter, "Gross morphology and fiber geometry of the heart," in *Handbook of Physiology: The Cardiovascular System* (B. Bethesda, ed.), vol. 1, pp. 61–112, American Physiology Society, 1979.

[4] F. H. Netter, *Farbatlanten der Medizin*, vol. 1. Georg Thieme Verlag, 1990.

[5] G.-R. Li, J. Feng, L. Yue, and M. Carrier, "Transmural heterogeneity of action potentials and I_{to1} in myocytes isolated from the human right ventricle," *Am. J. Physiol.*, vol. 275, pp. H369–H377, 1998.

[6] R. Cotran, V. Kumar, and T. Collins, *Robbins Pathologic Basis of Disease.* W. B. Saunders Company, 6 ed., 1999.

[7] M. A. Fallert, M. S. Mirotznik, S. W. Downing, E. B. Savage, K. R. Foster, M. E. Josephson, and D. K. Bogen, "Myocardial electrical impedance mapping of ischemic sheep hearts and healing aneurysms," *Circulation*, vol. 87, pp. 199–207, 1993.

[8] H.-H. Ebert, *Der EKG Lotse.* Georg Thieme Verlag, 2001.

[9] A. L. Hodgkin and A. F. Huxley, "A quantitative description of membrane current and its application to conduction and excitation in nerve," *J. Physiol.*, vol. 177, pp. 500–544, 1952.

[10] R. S. MacLeod and D. H. Brooks, "Recent progress in inverse problems of electrocardiography," *IEEE Eng. Med. Biol.*, vol. 17, no. 1, pp. 73–83, 1998.

[11] O. Skipa, *Linear inverse problem of electrocardiography: epicardial potentials and transmembrane voltages.* Helmesverlag Karlsruhe, 2004.

[12] J. Malmivuo and R. Plonsey, *Bioelectromagnetism - principles and applications of bioelectric and biomagnetic fields.* Oxford University Press, New York, 1995.

[13] R. Schmidt and G. Thews, *Physiologie des Menschen*. Springer-Verlag, 1997.

[14] U. J. Haag, O. M. Hess, S. E. Maier, M. Jakob, K. Liu, D. Meier, R. Jenni, P. Boesinger, M. Anliker, and H. P. Krayenbuehl, "Left ventricular wall thickness measurements by magnetic resonance: a validation study," *Int. J. Cardiac Imaging*, vol. 7, pp. 31–41, 1991.

[15] R. Klinge, *Das Elektrokardiogramm: Leitfaden für Ausbildung und Anwendung*. Georg Thieme Verlag, 1992.

[16] D. D. Streeter, jr. and D. L. Bassett, "An engineering analysis of myocardial fiber orientation in pig's left ventricle in systole," *Anatomical Record*, vol. 155, pp. 503–511, 1966.

[17] S. Silbernagl and A. Despopoulos, *Taschenatlas der Physiologie*. Georg Thieme Verlag, 2001.

[18] F. L. Burton and S. M. Cobbe, "Dispersion of ventricular repolarization and refractory period," *Cardiovasc. Res.*, vol. 50, pp. 10–23, 2001.

[19] C. Antzelevitch, S. Sicouri, S. H. Litovsky, A. Lukas, S. C. Krishman, J. M. Di Diego, G. A. Gintant, and D. W. Liu, "Heterogeneity within the ventricular wall: electrophysiology and pharmacology of epicardial, endocardial, and M-cells," *Circ. Res.*, vol. 69, pp. 1427–1449, 1991.

[20] C. Antzelevitch and J. Fish, "Electrical heterogeneity within the ventricular wall," *Basic Res. Cardiol.*, vol. 96, pp. 517–527, 2001.

[21] C. E. Conrath, R. Wilders, R. Coronel, J. M. de Bakker, P. Taggart, J. R. de Groot, and T. Opthof, "Intercellular coupling through gap junctions masks m cells in the human heart," *Cardiovasc Res.*, vol. 62, no. 2, pp. 407–414, 2004.

[22] K. H. W. J. ten Tusscher, D. Noble, P. J. Noble, and A. V. Panfilov, "A model for human ventricular tissue," *Am. J. Physiol.*, vol. 286, pp. H1573–H1589, 2004.

[23] G. Seemann, F. B. Sachse, D. L. Weiss, and O. Dössel, "Investigating heterogeneity in human heart with simulated transmural electrocardiograms," *Int J Bioelectromagnetism*, vol. 5, pp. 177–178, 2003.

[24] M. J. Janse, E. A. Sosunov, R. Coronel, T. Opthof, E. P. Anyukhovsky, J. M. T. de Bakker, A. N. Plotnikov, I. N. Shlapakova, P. Danilo, J. G. P. Tijssen, and M. R. Rosen, "Repolarization gradients in the canine left ventricle before and after induction of short-term cardiac memory," *Circ.*, vol. 112, no. 12, pp. 1711–1718, 2005.

[25] K. R. Laurita, S. D. Girouard, and D. S. Rosenbaum, "Modulation of ventricular repolarization by a premature stimulus: Role of epicardial dispersion of repolarization kinetics demonstrated by optical mapping of the intact guinea pig heart," *Circ. Res.*, vol. 79, pp. 493–503, 1996.

[26] J. W. Dean and M. J. Lab, "Regional changes in ventricular excitability during load manipulation of the in situ pig heart," *J Physiol*, vol. 429, pp. 387–400, 1990.

[27] M. Restivo, E. B. Caref, D. O. Kozhevnikov, and N. El-Sherif, "Spatial dispersion of repolarization is a key factor in the arrhythmogenicity of long qt syndrome," *J. Cardiovasc. Electrophys.*, vol. 15, pp. 323–331, 2004.

[28] J. M. Di Diego, Z. Q. Sun, and C. Antzelevitch, "I_{to} and action potential notch are smaller in left vs. right canine ventricular epicardium," *Am. J. Physiol.*, vol. 271, pp. 548–561, 1996.

[29] P. G. Volders, K. R. Sipido, E. Carmeliet, R. L. Spatjens, H. J. Wellens, and M. A. Vos, "Repolarizing K^+ currents I_{to1}, and I_{Ks} are larger in right than left canine ventricular myocardium," *Circ.*, vol. 99, pp. 206–210, 1999.

[30] E. Wettwer, G. J. Amos, H. Posival, and U. Ravens, "Transient outward current in human ventricular myocytes of subepicardial and subendocardial origin," *Circ. Res.*, vol. 75, pp. 473–482, 1994.

[31] D. L. Weiss, G. Seemann, D. U. J. Keller, D. Farina, F. B. Sachse, and O. Doessel, "Modeling of heterogeneous electrophysiology in the human heart with respect to ECG genesis," in *Proc. Computers in Cardiology*, 2007. in Press.

[32] A. van Oosterom, "Genesis of the T wave as based on an equivalent surface source model," *J. Electrocardiol.*, vol. 34, no. Suppl, pp. 217–27, 2001.

[33] A. van Oosterom and T. Oostendorp, "ECGSim: an interactive tool for studying the genesis of qrst forms," *Heart*, vol. 90, pp. 165–168, 2004.

[34] D. B. Geselowitz, "On the theory of the electrocardiogram," *Proc. of the IEEE*, vol. 77, pp. 857–876, June 1989.

[35] J. G. Stinstra, B. Hopenfeld, and R. S. Macleod, "On the passive cardiac conductivity," *Ann Biomed Eng*, vol. 33, no. 12, 2005.

[36] D. Farina and O. Dössel, "Influence of cardiac activity in midmyocardial cells on resulting ECG: Simulation study," in *Biomedizinische Technik 51(1)*, 2006. accepted.

[37] M. Jessup and S. Bronzena, "Heart failure," *N. Eng. J. Med.*, vol. 348, pp. 2007–2018, 2003.

[38] B.-D. Gonska and R. Heinecker, *EKG in Klinik und Praxis.* Georg Thieme Verlag, 1999.

[39] M. Glas, "Segmentation des Visible Man Datensatzes," Master's thesis, Universität Karlsruhe (TH), Institut für Biomedizinische Technik, June 1996. Diploma Thesis.

[40] F. B. Sachse, C. D. Werner, M. H. Stenroos, R. F. Schulte, P. Zerfass, and O. Dössel, "Modeling the anatomy of the human heart using the cryosection images of the Visible Female dataset," in *Proc. Third Users Conference of the National Library of Medicine's Visible Human Project*, (Bethesda, USA), 2000.

[41] S. Barros, N. S. Couto, F. B. Sachse, C. D. Werner, and G. Seemann, "Segmentation and tissue-classification of the visible female dataset - thoracic muscles, bones and blood vessels," in *Biomedizinische Technik*, vol. 46-1, pp. 510–511, Sep. 2001.

[42] J. C. Russ, *The image processing handbook.* CRC Press, 2 ed., 1995.

[43] F. B. Sachse, *Modelle des menschlichen Körpers zur Berechnung von physikalischen Feldern.* Shaker Verlag Aachen, 1998.

[44] P. Zerfass, F. B. Sachse, C. D. Werner, and O. Dössel, "Deformation of surface nets for interactive segmentation of tomographic data," in *Biomedizinische Technik*, vol. 45-1, pp. 483–484, Sep. 2000.

[45] N. H. Busch, F. B. Sachse, C. D. Werner, and O. Dössel, "Segmentation klinischer vierdimensionaler magnetresonanztomographischer Aufnahmen mittels Aktiver Kontur Modelle und haptischer Interaktion," in *Biomedizinische Technik*, vol. 43-1, pp. 526–529, Sep. 1998.

[46] L. Thomas, F. B. Sachse, C. D. Werner, and O. Dössel, "Topologisch veränderbare dreidimensionale Aktive Konturen in der medizinischen Bildverarbeitung," in *Biomedizinische Technik*, vol. 45-1, pp. 509–510, Sep. 2000.

[47] Y. Shang and O. Dössel, "Landmarking method of 3D surface models for construction of 4D cardiac shape model," in *Biomedizinische Technik*, vol. 48-1, pp. 124–125, 2003.

[48] Y. Shang and O. Dössel, "Construction of cardiac anatomical models using deformable model methods," in *Bildverarbeitung für die Medizin 2004*, (Berlin, Germany), pp. 209–213, Feb. 2004.

[49] Y. Shang and O. Dössel, "Statistical 3D shape-model guided segmentation of cardiac images," in *Proc. Computers in Cardiology*, (Chicago, USA), Oct. 2004.

[50] R. Plonsey and R. C. Barr, "Mathematical modeling of electrical activity of the heart," *J. Electrocardiol.*, vol. 20, no. 3, pp. 219–226, 1987.

[51] R. H. Mitchell, A. H. Bailey, and J. Anderson, "Cellular automaton model of ventricular fibrillation," *IEEE Trans. Biomed. Eng.*, vol. 39, no. 3, pp. 253–259, 1992.

[52] M. Lorange and R. M. Gulrajani, "A computer heart model incorporating anisotropic propagation," *J. Electrocardiol.*, vol. 26, no. 4, pp. 245–261, 1993.

[53] C. W. Zemlin and A. V. Panfilov, "Spiral waves in excitable media with negative restitution," *Phys. Rev.*, vol. 63, 2001.

[54] D. Hayn, *Ein Finite Elemente Herzmodell.* Graz University of Technology, 2002.

[55] B. He, G. Li, and X. Zhang, "Noninvasive imaging of cardiac transmembrane potentials within three-dimensional myocardium by means of a realistic geometry anisotropic heart model," *IEEE Trans. Biomed. Eng.*, vol. 50, no. 10, pp. 1190–1202, 2003.

[56] R. A. FitzHugh, "Impulses and physiological states in theoretical models of nerve membran," *Biophys. J.*, vol. 1, pp. 445–466, 1961.

[57] D. L. Weiß, G. Seemann, F. B. Sachse, and O. Dössel, "Investigation of electrophysiological heterogeneity and anisotropy across the human ventricular wall," in *Biomedizinische Technik*, vol. 48-1, pp. 228–229, 2003.

[58] G. Seemann, *Modeling of electrophysiology and tension development in the human heart.* PhD thesis, Institut f§r Biomedizinische Technik, UniversitŁtsverlag Karlsruhe ISBN 3-937300-66-X, 2005.

[59] D. L. Weiss, G. Seemann, F. B. Sachse, and O. Dössel, "Modelling of the short QT syndrome in a heterogeneous model of the human ventricular wall," *Europace*, vol. 7S2, pp. 105–117, 2005.

[60] D. Noble, "A modification of the Hodgkin-Huxley equation applicable to Purkinje fibre action and pacemaker potentials," *J. Physiol.*, vol. 160, pp. 317–352, 1962.

[61] R. E. McAllister, D. Noble, and R. W. Tsien, "Reconstruction of the electrical activitity of cardiac Purkinje fibres," *J. Physiol.*, vol. 251, pp. 1–59, 1975.

[62] G. W. Beeler and H. Reuter, "Reconstruction of the action potential of ventricular myocardial fibres," *J. Physiol.*, vol. 268, pp. 177–210, 1977.

[63] K. Yanagihara, A. Noma, and H. Irisawa, "Reconstruction of sinoatrial node pacemaker potential based on the voltage-clamp experiments," *Jpn. J. Physiol.*, vol. 30, pp. 841–857, 1980.

[64] D. G. Bristow and J. W. Clark, "A mathematical model of primary pacemaker cell in SA node of the heart," *Am. J. Physiol.*, vol. 243, no. 2, pp. H207–H218, 1982.

[65] D. G. Bristow and J. W. Clark, "A mathematical model of the vagally driven primary pacemaker," *Am. J. Physiol.*, vol. 244, no. 1, pp. H150–H161, 1983.

[66] D. Noble and S. J. Noble, "A model of sino-atrial node electrical activity based on a modification of the DiFrancesco-Noble (1984) equations," *Proc. R. Soc. Lond. B. Biol. Sci.*, vol. 222, pp. 295–304, 1984.

[67] D. DiFrancesco and D. Noble, "A model of cardiac electrical activity incorporating ionic pumps and concentration changes," *Phil. Trans. R. Soc. Lond.*, vol. 307, pp. 353–398, 1985.

[68] D. W. Hilgemann and D. Noble, "Excitation-contraction coupling and extracellular calcium transients in rabbit atrium: Reconstruction of basic cellular mechanisms," *Proc. R. Soc. Lond.*, vol. 230, pp. 163–205, 1987.

[69] Y. E. Earm and D. Noble, "A model of single atrial cell: Relation between calcium current and calcium release," *Proc. R. Soc. Lond.*, vol. 240, pp. 83–96, 1990.

[70] C.-H. Luo and Y. Rudy, "A model of the ventricular cardiac action potential," *Circ. Res.*, vol. 68, no. 6, pp. 1501–1526, 1991.

[71] C.-H. Luo and Y. Rudy, "A dynamic model of the ventricular cardiac action potential: I. Simulations of ionic currents and concentration changes," *Circ. Res.*, vol. 74, no. 6, pp. 1071–1096, 1994.

[72] C.-H. Luo and Y. Rudy, "A dynamic model of the ventricular cardiac action potential: II. Afterdepolarizations, triggered activity, and potentiation," *Circ. Res.*, vol. 74, no. 6, pp. 1097–1113, 1994.

[73] S. S. Demir, J. W. Clark, C. R. Murphey, and W. R. Giles, "A mathematical model of a rabbit sinoatrial node cell," *Am. J. Physiol.*, vol. 35, pp. 832–852, 1994.

[74] S. Dokos, B. G. Celler, and N. H. Lovell, "Vagal control of sinoatrial rhythm: A mathematical model," *J. Theor. Biol.*, vol. 182, pp. 21–44, Sep. 1996.

[75] D. S. Lindblad, C. R. Murphey, J. W. Clark, and W. R. Giles, "A model of the action potential and underlying membrane currents in a rabbit atrial cell," *Am. J. Physiol.*, vol. 271, no. 4 Pt 2, pp. H1666–H1696, 1996.

[76] S. S. Demir, B. O'Rourke, G. F. Tomaselli, E. Marbán, and R. L. Winslow, "Action potential variation in canine ventricle: A modeling study," in *Proc. Computers in Cardiology*, vol. 23, pp. 221–224, 1996.

[77] M. Courtemanche, R. J. Ramirez, and S. Nattel, "Ionic mechanisms underlying human atrial action potential properties: Insights from a mathematical model," *Am. J. Physiol.*, vol. 275, no. 44, pp. H301–H321, 1998.

[78] A. Nygren, C. Fiset, L. Firek, J. W. Clark, D. S. Lindblad, R. B. Clark, and W. R. Giles, "Mathematical model of an adult human atrial cell," *Circ. Res.*, vol. 82, pp. 63–81, 1998.

[79] M. S. Jafri, J. J. Rice, and R. L. Winslow, "Cardiac Ca^{2+} dynamics: The roles of ryanodine receptor adapation and sarcoplasmic reticulum load," *Biophysical J.*, vol. 74, pp. 1149–1168, Mar. 1998.

[80] D. Noble, A. Varghese, P. Kohl, and P. Noble, "Improved guinea-pig ventricular cell model incorporating a diadic space, I_{Kr} and I_{Ks}, and length- and tension-dependend processes," *Can. J. Cardiol.*, vol. 14, pp. 123–134, Jan. 1998.

[81] L. Priebe and D. J. Beuckelmann, "Simulation study of cellular electric properties in heart failure," *Circ. Res.*, vol. 82, pp. 1206–1223, 1998.

[82] S. S. Demir, J. W. Clark, and W. R. Giles, "Parasympatheticc modulation of sinoatrial node pacemaker activity in rabbit heart: A unifying model," *Am. J. Physiol.*, vol. 276, pp. H2221–H2244, 1999.

[83] R. L. Winslow, J. J. Rice, S. Jafri, E. Marbán, and B. O'Rourke, "Mechanisms of altered excitation-contraction coupling in canine tachycardia-induced heart failure, II model studies," *Circ. Res.*, vol. 84, pp. 571–586, 1999.

[84] R. J. Ramirez, S. Nattel, and M. Courtemanche, "Mathematical analysis of canine atrial action potentials: Rate, regional factors, and electrical remodeling," *Am. J. Physiol.*, vol. 279, pp. H1767–H1785, 2000.

[85] H. Zhang, A. V. Holden, I. Kodama, H. Honjo, M. Lei, T. Varghese, and M. R. Boyett, "Mathematical models of action potentials in the periphery and center of the rabbit sinoatrial node," *Am. J. Physiol.*, vol. 279, no. 1, pp. 397–421, 2000.

[86] M. R. Boyett, H. Zhang, A. Garny, and A. V. Holden, "Control of the pacemaker activity of the sinoatrial node by intracellular Ca^{2+}. Experiments and modelling," *Phil. Trans. R. Soc. London*, vol. 359, pp. 1091–1110, 2001.

[87] S. V. Pandit, R. B. Clark, W. R. Giles, and S. S. Demir, "A mathematical model of action potential heterogeneity in adult left ventricular myocytes," *Biophys. J.*, vol. 81, pp. 3029–3051, 2001.

[88] J. L. Puglisi and D. M. Bers, "LabHEART: An interactive computer model of rabbit ventricular myocyte ion channels and Ca transport," *Am. J. Physiol.*, vol. 281, pp. C2049–C2060, 2001.

[89] J. Kneller, R. J. Ramirez, D. Chartier, M. Courtemanche, and S. Nattel, "Time-dependent transients in an ionically based mathematical model of the canine atrial action potential," *Am. J. Physiol.*, vol. 282, pp. H1437–H1451, 2002.

[90] Y. Kurata, I. Hisatome, S. Imanishi, and T. Shibamoto, "Dynamical description of sinoatrial node pacemaking: Improved mathematical model for primary pacemaking cells," *Am. J. Physiol.*, vol. 283, pp. H2074–H2101, 2002.

[91] O. Bernus, R. Wilders, C. W. Zemlin, H. Verschelde, and A. V. Panfilov, "A computationally efficient electrophysiological model of human ventricular cells," *Am. J. Physiol.*, vol. 282, pp. H2296–H2308, 2002.

[92] N. H. Lovell, S. L. Cloherty, B. G. Celler, and S. Dokos, "A gradient model of cardiac pacemaking myocytes," *Progress in Biophysics and Molecular Biology*, vol. 85, no. 2-3, pp. 301–323, 2004.

[93] V. Iyer, R. Mazhari, and R. L. Winslow, "A computational model of the human left-ventricular epicardial myocyte," *Biophys. J.*, vol. 87, no. 3, pp. 1507–1525, 2004.

[94] S. Gabriel, R. W. Lau, and C. Gabriel, "The dielectric properties of biological tissues: II. measurements in the frequency range 10 hz to 20 ghz," *Phys. Med. Biol.*, vol. 41, pp. 2251–2269, 1996.

[95] Y. Rudy and R. Plonsey, "The eccentric spheres model as the basis for a study of the role of geometry and inhomogeneities in electrocardiography," *IEEE Trans Biomed Eng*, vol. 26, no. 7, pp. 392–399, 1979.

[96] M. Sadiku, *Numerical Techniques in Electromagnetics.* CRC Press, 2000.

[97] J. F. Thompson, B. K. Soni, and N. P. Weatherill, eds., *Handbook of Grid Generation.* CRC Press, 1999.

[98] M. Potse, B. Dubé, J. Richter, A. Vinet, and R. M. Gulrajani, "A comparison of monodomain and bidomain reaction-diffusion models for action potential propagation in the human heart," *IEEE Trans Biomed Eng*, vol. 53, no. 12, pp. 2425–2435, 2006.

[99] I. N. Bronstein and K. A. Semendjajew, *Taschenbuch der Mathematik.* Verlag Nauka, Moskau, 1985.

[100] G. H. Golub and C. F. V. Loan, *Matrix Computations.* The Johns Hopkins University Press, 1996.

[101] J. S. Hadamard, "Sur les problèmes aux dérivées partielles et leur signification physique," *Princeton University Bulletin*, vol. 13, pp. 49–52, 1902.

[102] P. C. Hansen, *Rank-deficient and discrete ill-posed problems: Numerical aspects of linear inversion.* SIAM, 1998.

[103] D. Brooks and R. MacLeod, "Electrical imaging of the heart," *IEEE Sign. Proc. Mag.*, vol. 14, pp. 24–42, 1997.

[104] R. Gulrajani, R. Roberge, and P. Savard, "The inverse problem of electrocardiography," in *Comprehensive Electrocardiology* (P. Macfarlane and T.T.V.Lawrie, eds.), vol. 1, pp. 237–288, Pergamon Press, 1989.

[105] O. Dössel, "Inverse problem of electro- and magnetocardiography: Review and recent progress," *IJBEM*, vol. 2, no. 2, 2002.

[106] A. J. Pullan, L. K. Cheng, M. P. Nash, C. P. Bradley, and D. J. Paterson, "Noninvasive electrical imaging of the heart: Theory and model development," *Ann. Biomed. Eng.*, vol. 29, no. 10, pp. 817–836, 2001.

[107] P. Franzone, B. Taccardi, and C. Viganotti, "An approach to inverse calculation of epicardial potentials from body surface maps," *Adv. Cardiol.*, vol. 21, pp. 50–54, 1978.

[108] R. Barr and M. Spach, "Inverse calculation of QRS-T epicardial potentials from body surface potential distributions for normal and ectopic beats in the intact dog," *Circ. Res.*, vol. 42, pp. 661–675, 1978.

[109] E. Downar, I. Parson, L. Mickleborough, D. Cameron, L. Yao, and M. Waxman, "On-line epicardial mapping of intraoperative ventricular arrhythmias: initial clinical experience," *J. Am. Coll. Cardiol.*, vol. 4, pp. 703–714, 1984.

[110] L. Green, B. Taccardi, P. Ershler, and R. Lux, "Epicardial potential mapping. effects of conducting media on isopotential and isochrone distributions," *Circ.*, vol. 84, pp. 2513–2521, 1991.

[111] M. S. Fuller, G. Sándor, B. Punske, B. Taccardi, R. S. MacLeod, P. R. Ershler, L. S. Green, and R. L. Lux, "Estimates of repolarization dispersion from electrocardiographic measurements," *Circ.*, vol. 102, pp. 685–691, 2000.

[112] R. N. Ghanem, P. Jia, C. Ramanathan, K. Ryu, A. Markowitz, and Y. Rudy, "Noninvasive electrocardiographic imaging (ECGI): Comparison to intraoperative mapping in patients," *Heart Rhythm*, vol. 2, no. 4, pp. 339–354, 2005.

[113] J. de Bakker, M. Janse, J. van Capelle, and D. Durrer, "Endocardial mapping by simultaneous recording of endocardial electrograms during cardiac surgery for ventricular aneurysm," *J. Am. Coll. Cardiol.*, vol. 2, pp. 947–953, 1983.

[114] D. S. Khoury, B. Taccardi, R. L. Lux, P. R. Ershler, and Y. Rudy, "Reconstruction of endocardial potentials and activation sequences from intracavitary probe measurements," *Circ.*, vol. 91, pp. 845–863, 1995.

[115] D. S. Khoury, K. L. Berrier, S. M. Badruddin, and W. A. Zoghbi, "Three-dimensional electrophysiological imaging of the intact canine left ventricle using a noncontact multielectrode cavitary probe: Study of sinus, paced, and spontaneous premature beats," *Circ.*, vol. 97, pp. 399–409, 1998.

[116] O. Skipa, M. Nalbach, F. Sachse, C. Werner, and O. Dössel, "Transmembrane potential reconstruction in anisotropic heart model," *IJBEM*, vol. 4, pp. 17–18, 2002.

[117] B. Messnarz, B. Tilg, R. Modre, G. Fischer, and F. Hanser, "A new spatiotemporal regularization approach for reconstruction of cardiac transmembrane potential patterns," *IEEE Trans. Biomed. Eng.*, vol. 51, no. 2, pp. 273–281, 2004.

[118] B. Messnarz, M. Seger, R. Modre, G. Fischer, F. Hanser, and B. Tilg, "A comparison of noninvasive reconstruction of epicardial versus transmembrane potentials in consideration of the space," *IEEE Trans. Biomed. Eng.*, vol. 51, no. 9, pp. 1609–1618, 2004.

[119] G. Huiskamp and A. van Oosterom, "The depolarization sequence of the human heart surface computed from measured body surface potentials," *IEEE Trans. Biomed. Eng.*, vol. 35, no. 12, pp. 1047–1058, 1988.

[120] B. Tilg, R. Modre, F. Hanser, B. Messnarz, M. Schocke, C. Kremser, T. Berger, F. Hintringer, and F. X. Roithinger, "Model-based imaging of cardiac electrical excitation in humans," *IEEE Trans. Med. Im.*, vol. 21, no. 9, pp. 1031–1039, 2001.

[121] R. Modre, B. Tilg, G. Fischer, and P. Wach, "Noninvasive myocardial activation time imaging: A novel inverse algorithm applied to clinical ECG mapping data," *IEEE Trans. Biomed. Eng.*, vol. 49, no. 10, pp. 1153–1161, 2002.

[122] T. Berger, G. Fischer, B. Pfeifer, R. Modre, F. Hanser, T. Trieb, F. X. Roithinger, M. Stuehlinger, O. Pachinger, B. Tilg, and F. Hintringer, "Single-beat noninvasive imaging of cardiac electrophysiology of ventricular pre-excitation," *J. Am. Coll. Cardiol.*, vol. 48, no. 10, pp. 2045–2052, 2006.

[123] C. Ramanathan, R. N. Ghanem, P. Jia, K. Ryu, and Y. Rudy, "Noninvasive electrocardiographic imaging for cardiac electrophysiology and arrhythmia," *Nature Med.*, vol. 10, no. 4, pp. 422–428, 2004.

[124] O. Dössel and F. R. Schneider, "The nullspace of electrocardiography," *Biomedizinische Technik*, vol. 42-1, pp. 37–40, 1997.

[125] D. Colton, H. W. Engl, A. K. Louis, J. R. McLaughlin, and W. Rundell, eds., *Surveys on solution methods for inverse problems.* Springer Verlag Austria, 2000.

[126] E. Anderson, Z. Bai, C. Bischof, S. Blackford, J. Demmel, J. Dongarra, J. D. Croz, A. Greenbaum, S. Hammarling, A. McKenney, and D. Sorensen, *LAPACK Users' Guide.* SIAM, 3 ed., 1999.

[127] A. N. Tikhonov and V. Y. Arsenin, *Solutions of ill-posed problem.* Winston&Sons, New York, 1977.

[128] P. C. Hansen, "The L-curve and its use in the numerical treatment of inverse problems," in *Computational inverse problems in electrocardiography*, ch. 4, pp. 119–142, WIT Press, Advances in Computational Bioengineering, 2001.

[129] P. C. Hansen and D. P. O'Leary, "The use of L-curve in the regularization of discrete ill-posed problems," *SIAM J. Sci. Comput.*, vol. 14, no. 6, pp. 1487–1503, 1993.

[130] M. Foster, "An application of the Wiener-Kolmogorov smoothing theory to matrix inversion," *J. Soc. Ind. Appl. Math.*, vol. 9/3, pp. 387–392, 1961.

[131] D. D. Jackson, "The use of *a priori* data to resolve non-uniqueness in linear inversion," *Geophys. J. R. astr. Soc.*, vol. 57, pp. 137–157, 1979.

[132] J. N. Franklin, "Well-posed stochastic extension of ill-posed problems," *J. Math. Anal. Appl.*, vol. 31, pp. 682–716, 1970.

[133] A. van Oosterom, "The use of the spatial covariance in computing pericardial potentials," *IEEE Trans. Biomed. Eng.*, vol. 46, no. 7, pp. 778–787, 1999.

[134] D. Farina, Y. Jiang, O. Skipa, O. Dössel, C. Kaltwasser, and W. R. Bauer, "The use of the simulation results as a priori information to solve the inverse problem of electrocardiography for a patient," *Proc Computers in Cardiography*, pp. 571–574, 2005.

[135] Y. Jiang, "Implementation of a stochastic regularization method to solve the inverse problem of electrocardiography," Master's thesis, Institut für Biomedizinische Technik, Universität Karlsruhe (TH), 2005.

[136] Y. Serinagaoglu, D. H. Brooks, and R. S. MacLeod, "Bayesian solutions and performance analysis in bioelectric inverse problems," *IEEE Trans. Biomed. Eng.*, vol. 52, no. 6, pp. 1009–1020, 2005.

[137] Y. Serinagaoglu, D. H. Brooks, and R. S. MacLeod, "Improved performance of bayesian solutions for inverse electrocardiography using multiple information sources," *IEEE Trans. Biomed. Eng.*, vol. 53, no. 10, pp. 2024–2034, 2006.

[138] Y. Jiang, D. Farina, C. Kaltwasser, O. Dössel, and W. R. Bauer, "Modeling and reconstruction of myocardial infarction," in *Biomedizinische Technik*, 2006.

[139] Y. Jiang, D. Farina, and O. Dössel, "An improved spatio-temporal maximum a posteriori approach to solve the inverse problem of electrocardiography," in *Biomedizinische Technik*, 2007.

[140] Y. Jiang, D. Farina, and O. Dössel, "Reconstruction of myocardial infarction using the improved spatio-temporal map-based regularization," in *The 6th International Symposium on Noninvasive Functional Source Imaging of the Brain and Heart and the International Conference on Functional Biomedical Imaging*, 2007.

[141] D. Calvetti, B. Lewis, and L. Reichel, "GMRes, L-curves, and discrete ill-posed problems," *BIT*, vol. 42, no. 1, pp. 44–65, 2002.

[142] C. Ramanathan, P. Jia, R. Ghanem, D. Calvetti, and Y. Rudy, "Noninvasive electrocardiographic imaging (ECGI): Application of the generalized minimal residual (GMRes) method," *Ann. Biomed. Eng.*, vol. 31, no. 8, pp. 981–994, 2003.

[143] W. Arnoldi, "The principle of minimized iterations in the solution of the matrix eigenvalue problem," *Quart. Appl. Math.*, vol. 9, pp. 17–29, 1951.

[144] D. Calvetti, L. Reichel, and Q. Zhang, "Iterative solution methods for large linear discrete ill-posed problems," *Appl. Comput. Control, Signals and Circuits*, vol. 1, pp. 313–367, 1999.

[145] R. Barrett, M. Berry, T. F. Chan, J. Demmel, J. Donato, J. Dongarra, V. Eijkhout, R. Pozo, C. Romine, and H. V. der Vorst, *Templates for the Solution of Linear Systems: Building Blocks for Iterative Methods, 2nd Edition.* Philadelphia, PA: SIAM, 1994.

[146] F. Greensite and G. Huiskamp, "An improved method for estimating epicardial potentials from the body surface," *IEEE Trans. Biomed. Eng.*, vol. 45, pp. 98–104, 1998.

[147] F. B. Sachse, W. Bauer, O. Dössel, and M. Meesmann, "Lokale Charakterisierung der Repolarisation im ventrikulären Myokard ausgehend von extrakorporalen Multikanal-Elektrokardiogrammen," *Beschreibung des DFG-Projekts*, 2001.

[148] J. Frahm, A. Haase, and D. Matthaei, "Rapid NMR imaging of dynamic processes using the FLASH technique," *Magn. Reson. Med.*, vol. 3, no. 2, pp. 321–327, 1986.

[149] A. Haase, J. Frahm, D. Matthaei, W. Haenicke, and K. Merboldt, "FLASH imaging, rapid NMR imaging using low flip-angle pulses," *J. Magn. Reson.*, vol. 67, no. 2, pp. 258–266, 1986.

[150] W. Press, S. Teukolsky, W. Vetterling, and B. Flannery, *Numerical recipes in C.* Cambridge University Press, 1991.

[151] L. Fainzilberg, "Restoration of a standard sample of cyclic waveforms with the use of the Hausdorff metric in a phase space," *Cybernetics and Systems Analysis*, vol. 39, no. 3, pp. 338–344, 2003.

[152] A. Khawaja, S. Sanyal, and O. Dössel, "Temporal analysis of multi-channel QRS complexes using pca," *Biomedizinische Technik*, vol. 50, no. 1, pp. 277–278, 2005.

[153] A. Khawaja and O. Dössel, "A pca-based technique for qrs complex estimation," in *Proc. Computers in Cardiology*, vol. 32, pp. 747–750, 2005.

[154] S. Seitz, A. Khawaja, and O. Dössel, "PCA-based method for clustering T-Waves," in *Jahrestagung der Deutschen Gesellschaft für Biomedizinische Technik*, 2006.

[155] A. Khawaja and O. Dössel, "Predicting the QRS complex and detecting small changes using principal component analysis," *Biomed Tech.*, vol. 52, pp. 11–17, 2007.

[156] C. Werner, *Simulation der elektrischen Erregungsausbreitung in anatomischen Herzmodellen mit adaptiven Zellulaeren Automaten.* Tenea, Berlin, 2001.

[157] A. Kleber and C. Riegger, "Electrical constants of arterially perfused rabbit papillary muscle," *J. Physiol.*, vol. 385, pp. 307–324, 1987.

[158] O. Skipa, M. Nalbach, and O. Dössel, "The effect of cardiac anisotropy on the reconstruction of transmembrane voltages in the heart," in *Biomedizinische Technik*, vol. 48-1, pp. 472–473, 2003.

[159] *Image Processing Handbook.* CRC Press, 2 ed., 1995.

[160] "PhysioNet/Computers in Cardiology Challenge 2007: Electrocardiographic Imaging of Myocardial Infarction."

[161] D. Farina and O. Dössel, "Model-based approach to the localization of infarction," in *Proc. Computers in Cardiology*, 2007. in Press.

[162] W. T. Miller and D. B. Geselowitz, "Simulation studies of the electrocardiogram. II. Ischemia and infarction," *Circ. Res.*, vol. 43, pp. 315–323, 1978.

[163] B. Wohlfart, "A simple model for demonstration of STT-changes in ECG," *Europ. Heart J.*, vol. 8, pp. 409–416, 1987.

[164] B. Dubé, R. M. Gulrajani, M. Lorange, A. R. LeBlanc, J. Nasmith, and R. A. Nadeau, "A computer heart model incorporating anisotropic propagation. IV. Simulation of regional myocardial ischemia," *J. Electrocardiol.*, vol. 29, no. 2, pp. 91–103, 1996.

[165] F. Hanser, M. Seger, B. Tilg, R. Modre, G. Fischer, B. Messnarz, F. Hintringer, T. Berger, and F. X. Roithinger, "Influence of ischemic and infarcted tissue on the surface potential," in *Proc. Computers in Cardiology*, vol. 30, pp. 789–792, 2003.

[166] B. Dubé, R. M. Gulrajani, M. Lorange, A. R. LeBlanc, J. Nasmith, and R. A. Nadeau, "Simulation of ST segment changes during subendocardial ischemia using a realistic 3-D cardiac geometry," *IEEE Trans. Biomed. Eng.*, vol. 52, no. 5, pp. 799–807, 2005.

[167] R. Modre, M. Seger, G. Fischer, C. Hintermüller, D. Hayn, B. Pfeifer, F. Hanser, G. Schreier, and B. Tilg, "Cardiac anisotropy: Is it negligible regarding noninvasive activation time imaging?," *IEEE Trans. Biomed. Eng.*, vol. 53, pp. 569–580, April 2006.

[168] B. van Ginneken, A. F. Frangi, J. J. Staal, B. M. ter Haar Romeny, and M. A. Viergever, "Active shape model segmentation with optimal features," *IEEE Trans. Med. Imaging*, vol. 21, pp. 924–933, August 2002.

[169] G. Huiskamp and F. Greensite, "A new method for myocardial activation imaging," *IEEE Trans. Biomed. Eng.*, vol. 44, pp. 433–446, June 1997.

Danksagung

Mein besonderer Dank gilt Herrn Prof. Dr. rer. nat. Olaf Dössel für das große Interesse an dieser Arbeit und die jederzeit achtsame und kompetente Betreuung. Außerdem möchte ich mich für die Übernahme des Hauptreferats herzlich bedanken.

Herrn Prof. Dipl.-Ing. Dr. Bernhard Tilg danke ich für das Interesse an der Arbeit und die Übernahme des Korreferats.

Meinem Freund und ehemaligen Kollegen Herrn Dr.-Ing. Oleg Skipa möchte ich danken für die mehrjährige Zusammenarbeit und stetige Unterstützung. Auch Herrn Yuan Jiang danke ich für die effektive und freundschaftliche Zusammenarbeit. Meinen Kollegen Herrn Dr.-Ing. Gunnar Seemann und Herrn Daniel Weiß danke ich für ihre guten Ratschläge und Diskussionen.

Ich danke Herrn Prof. Dr. med. Wolfgang R. Bauer und Herrn Christoph Kaltwasser für das Überlassen der Messdaten und die freundliche Zusammenarbeit im Rahmen des gemeinsamen Projektes.

Herrn Frank Weber möchte ich danken für die große Hilfe bei der Korrektur dieser Arbeit.

Frau Rotraut Frech danke ich herzlich für ihre wertvolle Hilfe beim Erlernen der deutschen Sprache.

Nicht zuletzt möchte ich mich bei meiner Frau Maryna und meinem Sohn Sergej für ihre Geduld und stetig liebevolle Unterstützung bedanken, ohne den diese Arbeit nicht zustande gekommen wäre.

Printed in Dunstable, United Kingdom

91622768R00127